AN EASY-TO-FOLLOW PROGRAM FOR OVERCOMING
AND ITS PAIN THROUGH LOW-IMPACT EXERCISE

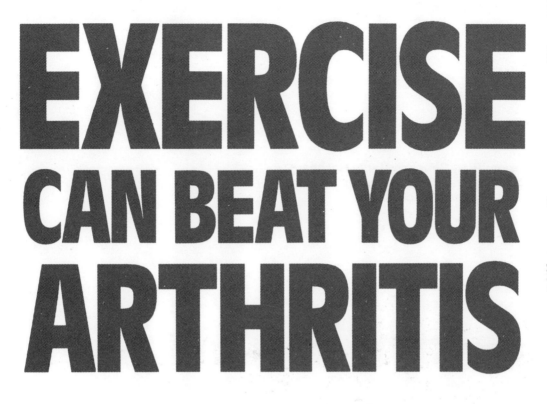

EXERCISE
CAN BEAT YOUR
ARTHRITIS

VALERIE SAYCE
IAN FRASER

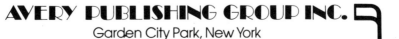

AVERY PUBLISHING GROUP INC.
Garden City Park, New York

The information and exercises presented in this book are based on the training, personal experience, and research of the authors. Because each person and situation is unique, the publisher and authors urge the reader to check with a qualified health professional before using any exercise where there is any question as to its appropriateness. It is a sign of wisdom, not cowardice, to seek a second or third opinion.

Cover Design: Rudy Shur and Martin Hochberg
Cover Photo: Central Reproduction and Photography
Typesetting: Multifacit Graphics, Inc.

Library of Congress Cataloging-in-Publication Data

Sayce, Valerie.
    Exercise can beat your arthritis.

    Bibliography: p.
    Includes index.
    1. Arthritis--Exercise therapy. I. Fraser,
Ian, 1936-   . II. Title.
RC933.S26 1989   616.7 ' 22062   89-249
ISBN 0-89529-392-7

Printed in the United States of America.

10 9 8 7 6 5 4 3 2 1

CONTENTS

ACKNOWLEDGMENTS

Our thanks are due to many people who helped or contributed to the book in their different ways.

Dr. Danny Lewis, Rheumatologist and Member of the Board of the Arthritis Foundation of Victoria, reviewed the exercise sequences and provided several helpful suggestions that, in the end, have made the book that much the better.

Jenny Davidson, the AFV's Programs Manager, drew generously from her expertise on many occasions during the book's embryonic and developmental phases; and she also carefully checked through manuscript and proofs.

Mary Balfour, until recently Chief Executive of the AFV, gave us ample encouragement to initiate the project and to keep it going when it might otherwise have waned.

All our models, themselves affected by arthritis of one kind or another, brimmed full of enthusiasm for the project right from the start. Without them and their keen involvement, no book would have been possible; so special thanks are due to Erna Attard, June Richards, Doris Morris, Gweneth Way Lee, Victor Wetherall, Sue Tardif, Mark Pace and Rikki Bewley.

Two senior Melbourne physiotherapists, Gabrielle Bortoluzzi (Box Hill Hospital) and Jill Exton (Children's Hospital), provided useful reactions and comments on the manuscript, and we are grateful to them, as we are to several other members of the physiotherapy profession who pointed us in the right direction.

Deborah Merritt, of Hawaii Therapeutic Exercise, took an early interest in *Exercise Beats Arthritis* during her successful visit to Australia for Arthritis Week '86. Since then, she has kept in touch with the book, offering constructive comments about the exercises. Deborah sees the book as being 'helpful to many people, not just those with arthritis'.

To our graphic artist, Judith Groenendijk, we also owe a vote of thanks. She was ever patient and flexible in looking at solutions to the design problems we inevitably posed. Flexibility and good vision were also attributes we found in abundance in our photographer, Roger Gould.

Sue Seagle did such an excellent job of typing the manuscript that it made the typesetter's task so much easier.

We are in debt to these and to many others for their help, encouragement and ideas — not least to the Arthritis Foundation of Victoria itself.

FOREWORD

There is nothing new about the importance of exercise for all people with arthritis. The problem has always been knowing how much to exercise, when to exercise and how not to overdo. Of course, there is the other problem — getting up the motivation to start and, more importantly, maintain an exercise program. This book is excellent in that it answers the first questions. More importantly, it presents a simple set of exercises which can be done by nearly everyone with arthritis in just a few minutes a day. The suggested routines are not complex. They do not need special equipment nor are they time consuming. In fact, they may seem so simple that they will be ignored for more complex, difficult or expensive routines. Don't be fooled; this is one time that simple and easy is best!! Our friends in Australia, the authors, have a great deal to teach us and have done so in an easy-to-master fashion.

The philosophy of this book mirrors our own. That is, people with arthritis must be responsible for their own day-to-day management. The more one can be in control of his or her life, the more one can master living with arthritis. The suggestions made by the authors are excellent. Of course, if you have any questions about your exercise program you should ask your physician or physical therapist. Better yet, take this book with you. Then you can choose to write any notes on changes or suggestions that they make.

All in all, this book should make an excellent addition to your arthritis self-help library. As they would say in Australia, "Well done, Mates!"

Dr. Kate Lorig
Senior Research Associate
Stanford Arthritis Center
Stanford University School of Medicine
Stanford, California

ABOUT THE AUTHORS

Valerie Sayce trained as a physiotherapist at the Lincoln Institute of Health Sciences. For some years now, she has been involved with land and water exercise programs. She conducts regular exercise and relaxation classes at the Arthritis Foundation and elsewhere in the community, and has played a key role in developing the Foundation's Water Exercise Recreation Program.

Her interest in exercise extends into exercise-stretch-relaxation classes for pregnant and post-natal women, and aerobic rhythm-exercise classes. She has also studied and taught Tai Chi—the Chinese art of moving meditation.

Educated in Scotland, *Ian Fraser* has worked in education and in publishing for over 20 years. He has written two English textbooks and numerous other handbooks for teachers. His varied experiences in the world of work have included teaching, educational research, personnel, college administration, radio and publishing, here and overseas. Exercise, he claims, is beating his osteoarthritis.

LEARN TO LIVE WITH IT

Arthritis and rheumatism are very general terms which cover a wide range of joint problems and other aches and pains. Most of us experience something of the kind at some time in our lives. It is only when the symptoms linger, or if they are particularly painful, that we seek advice and help from our doctor.

You may already have sought help. Perhaps you got good advice, or maybe you were told, 'Oh, you've just got a bit of arthritis. Here is something for the pain. Not much we can do — you'll just have to learn to live with it.'

This presents a rather hopeless picture, doesn't it? You think your pain and suffering have not been taken seriously. However, it is not true that nothing can be done. Think carefully about the words 'learn to live with it'. It is actually very good advice.

'Learning to live with it' does not mean that you withdraw from life for fear of doing anything that might aggravate your condition. This will only lead to your feeling miserable and sorry for yourself. Nor does it mean the other extreme of deliberately ignoring what your body is saying to you, in an attempt to maintain your normal high-powered lifestyle. Rather, you must find a balance whereby you *learn* to *live* with your arthritis. You learn to recognize, listen and respond to your body's signals.

A good starting point is to find out about the type of arthritis you have and what it is doing to your body. Become more aware, also, what your body is telling you: what makes you feel worse, what makes you feel better. And, above all, recognize there is a lot *you* can do to help yourself. The more understanding you have of your problem, the better you will be able to manage your arthritis. You can still lead a satisfying and enjoyable life.

So how can *Exercise Beats Arthritis* help you achieve this aim? Arthritis is primarily a disease which affects your joints and their support structures. Exercises use those joints and muscles, so it's in your power to work directly on your problems.

Different exercises have different purposes. For instance, some exercises are designed to strengthen your muscles, some are more effective in increasing the range of movement of your joints, and yet others improve your general fitness.

As you will find through reading this book and practicing the exercises, there are many ways in which exercises can have beneficial effects.

Exercise is one of the most useful and direct ways in which *you* can help minimize the pain and the limitations of arthritis. However, be careful what type of exercise you do. It is possible to make your problems worse with improper exercises. By working through this book, you will be able to develop an appropriate and beneficial exercise program *for you and your arthritis*.

WHAT IS ARTHRITIS?

The word 'arthritis' means literally inflammation of the joint. However, in general usage the term covers a multitude of problems affecting the joints, the muscles and the connective tissues of the body. There are over 100 different kinds of arthritis, but in this book we will discuss only the most common varieties.

If you are reading this book, you may have already been to your doctor who diagnosed your condition as arthritis; or maybe you just have a few aches and pains that you think might be arthritis.

What are the usual signs and symptoms of arthritis?

- Recurrent pain or tenderness in a joint
- Inability to move a joint normally
- Swelling, redness or heat in one or more joints
- Joint stiffness when you wake up in the morning
- Unexplained loss of weight, fever, weakness or fatigue, combined with joint pain.

If any of these symptoms lasts for more than two weeks, you should go and see your doctor who will be able to tell whether or not you have arthritis.

The various types of arthritis have specific effects on the different parts of the joint. You will understand more about your arthritis if you appreciate the function of the various structures within the normal joint.

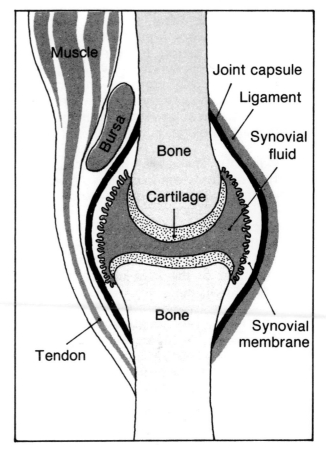

A normal joint

1. *Bones:* Two bones meet to form the joint. The ends of the bones are smooth and shaped to fit into each other. It is the shape of the bones which determines the type of movement in a joint.

2. *Cartilage:* The surfaces of the bones within the joint are covered by cartilage. This is a smooth tough elastic substance which cushions and protects the ends of the bones.

3. *Joint capsule:* Completely surrounding the joint and holding everything together is the tough fibrous joint capsule.

4. *Synovial membrane:* Lining the inner surface of the joint capsule is a thin membrane called the synovial membrane.

5. *Synovial fluid:* The synovial membrane secretes a very important fluid with a consistency similar to egg-white. During movement, this synovial fluid is squeezed between the joint surfaces and acts as a lubricant to ensure the smooth function of the joint. It also provides nourishment to the joint cartilage.

6. *Ligaments:* These are short fibrous cords which reinforce the joint capsule and help maintain the stability of the joint.

7. *Muscles:* The joint is moved by the muscles which pass over it. Muscle tissue is elastic so it can become shorter or longer. Movement of the joint occurs when the muscles contract.

8. *Tendons:* The muscles are usually attached to the bones by strong fibrous cords. These tendons are enclosed in a sheath which secretes synovial fluid to provide smooth movement.

9. *Bursa:* Near some joints there are small cushions between the bones and tendons or muscles. These bursae are small sacs, lined with synovial membrane and filled with synovial fluid.

RHEUMATOID ARTHRITIS

What picture comes into your mind when you think about someone suffering with arthritis? Many people have the idea that arthritis is a painful and crippling disease resulting in unsightly joint deformities, and that anyone who has arthritis is severely restricted in what they are able to do. The disease that they have in mind is rheumatoid arthritis. It is true that in its most severe form, or when it is not well managed, rheumatoid arthritis can result in very painful and badly damaged joints — and much suffering. However, for most people with rheumatoid arthritis, it's quite possible to lead a fairly normal life.

Rheumatoid arthritis is a widespread disease. It affects about 3% of the population, three-quarters of whom are women. Usually the disease begins in mid-life, but it can start at any age.

The course of the disease varies from person to person. In its mildest form, rheumatoid arthritis is an illness lasting only a few months and leaving no disability. Or it may come and go — with episodes of illness interspersed with periods of normal health.

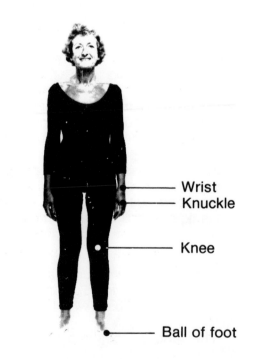

Wrist
Knuckle

Knee

Ball of foot

Common sites of rheumatoid arthritis

For most people, though, the disease progresses for a number of years with periods of flare-up and remission. The rate of progress is very variable. Fortunately, in most cases, the disease tends to burn itself out and after a time causes no further damage.

So what causes rheumatoid arthritis? What happens to your body? The exact cause is unknown, but it does involve the body's immune system which normally protects you from disease. In rheumatoid arthritis, it appears that some causative factor triggers your immune system to react against your own tissues — in particular the joints. The result is that the synovial membrane lining the inside of the joint becomes inflamed and enlarged.

This makes the joint warm, swollen and painful. The inflamed synovial tissue produces enzymes which are released into the joint. These cause more irritation and pain. Eventually the enzymes may eat away the structures inside the joint — cartilage, bone, ligaments — and this is what causes the permanent joint deformities.

Rheumatoid arthritis affects your whole body, not just your joints. It may cause inflammation in the muscles, tendons, lungs, skin, blood vessels, nerves and eyes. Many people with rheumatoid arthritis feel generally tired and run down. Loss of appetite and weight is common. Some people have a slight fever.

Any joint can be affected by rheumatoid arthritis, but usually the same joints on both sides of the body are involved, most commonly the wrists, knuckles, knees and the balls of the feet.

Treatment for rheumatoid arthritis reflects the variability of the disease and is really an individualized management program. It involves a combination of medication, rest, exercise, joint protection and, in extreme circumstances, surgery. Common sense, a positive attitude and understanding from others play a large part in a successful management program.

Exercise and Rheumatoid Arthritis

Rheumatoid arthritis requires a delicate balance of rest and activity. When your joints are hot, swollen and painful they need to be rested, although they should still be taken through their range of movement one or two

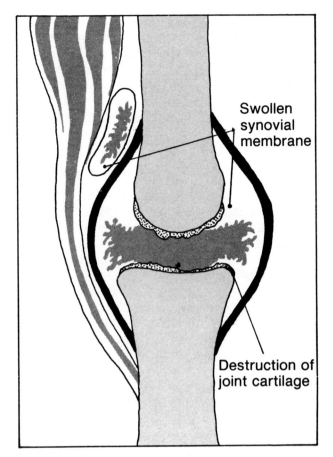

Effects of rheumatoid arthritis on a joint

times a day. At other times, regular exercise is essential in order to maintain the maximum function of joints and muscles.

This book gives you the opportunity to develop a suitable exercise program for your condition.

OSTEOARTHRITIS

How often do you hear someone complaining about an odd ache or pain and then dismissing it by saying, 'I must be getting old'? As everyone gets older, their joints show some signs of degeneration, although for the majority of people this causes little or no problem. When this process starts to produce pain, it is known by a number of names — osteoarthritis, osteoarthrosis, OA, degenerative joint disease, cervical spondylosis (in the neck), and lumbar spondylosis (in the lower back).

Osteoarthritis is a completely different condition to rheumatoid arthritis, although some people may have both. With osteoarthritis, only the joint itself is affected. Usually there is no inflammation. The main structure affected in osteoarthritis is the cartilage that covers the ends of the bones. It softens and becomes pitted and frayed, so movement is no longer smooth and easy. Cartilage has only a limited ability to heal itself since it does not have any blood supply.

With aging, the cartilage loses some of its resilience and is unable to absorb the same stresses as before. Gradually the cartilage is eroded, exposing the bone itself. In severe cases the destructive process can affect the underlying bony surfaces. Sometimes pieces of cartilage break off and float around in the joint. Moving an osteoarthritic joint can be very painful. Your body makes an effort to solve the problem by trying to increase the weight-bearing area of the joint. Bony spurs (called 'osteophytes') form in the places where the ligaments and joint capsule attach to the bone. These osteophytes can themselves cause problems, particularly in the spine.

But not everyone develops osteoarthritis, so there must be factors other than age which contribute to the breakdown of the cartilage. It's possible that some people are born with less resilient cartilage, or that their joints do not fit together very well, or maybe they move incorrectly. Osteoarthritis is much more likely to develop in joints that have been injured in some way — say, through a fracture or dislocation, or if they have been subjected to too much load.

Contrary to what you might think, vigorous use of a joint does not necessarily lead to osteoarthritis. This is because it is through activity that the synovial fluid, which lubricates and nourishes the joint, is squeezed into the cartilage; and this seems to counteract any damage which may be happening.

Effects of osteoarthritis on a joint

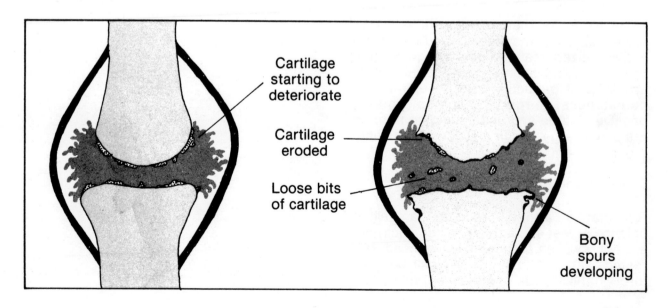

Cartilage starting to deteriorate

Cartilage eroded

Loose bits of cartilage

Bony spurs developing

Osteoarthritis can occur in any joint, but it is usually the joints under most stress which are commonly affected: hips, knees, neck, lower spine, base of the big toe and thumb, and the end joints of the fingers. Some people, more often women, develop a bony thickening at the end finger joints.

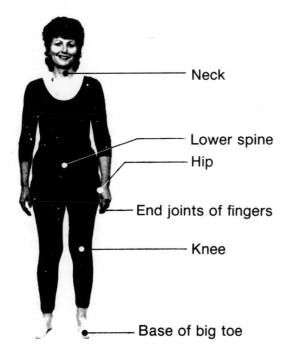

Common sites of osteoarthritis

Osteoarthritis is an ongoing degenerative condition, so treatment is aimed at relieving the symptoms and preventing further damage. Management involves a combination of exercise, rest, medication, weight control, comfort techniques, joint protection and, only if absolutely necessary, surgery.

You can obtain a lot of relief by sticking faithfully to your treatment program.

Exercise and Osteoarthritis

Regular and appropriate exercise is probably the best way to get relief from your osteoarthritis. As we have already mentioned, the cartilage is nourished when you move your joints. So keeping active helps prevent further degeneration. Exercise will also strengthen the muscles around the joint, providing it with greater support.

This does not mean that you should undertake a strenuous, exhausting exercise pro- gram, which will only cause more damage. Nor should you force yourself to exercise a very painful joint. Pain is a message from your body that something is wrong. You must take heed and rest the joint.

This book will help you to develop an exercise program suitable for your osteoarthritic joints.

ANKYLOSING SPONDYLITIS

Ankylosing spondylitis is not a common form of arthritis, but it is one in which exercise plays a key part. The main feature of ankylosing spondylitis is stiffness of the spine, which can become completely rigid if the disease is not properly managed.

Ankylosing spondylitis is more prevalent among men than women, and it usually affects younger people (15–25 years old). Very often, however, symptoms are not recognized as ankylosing spondylitis until the person is a bit older.

Ankylosing spondylitis is different from other arthritic conditions in that it affects structures outside the joint, rather than inside. It starts with inflammation of the ends of the ligaments where they attach to the bone. The joint most commonly involved is the sacroiliac joint, the joint between the bottom of the spine and the pelvis.

The first symptom of ankylosing spondylitis is usually stiffness and pain in the lower back. The inflammation gradually spreads to the joints further up the spine and may affect the attachment of the ribs to the spine. It may spread down to the hips, but only rarely are the other joints of the limbs involved.

The inflammation causes pain and stiffness, but this is not the end of the problem. After a while, bony outgrowths spread along the ligaments forming a solid bridge between the two bones. Obviously, this means that the joint cannot move. The only benefit is that it is no longer painful. This fusion of the joints of the spine is what leads to the rigid 'poker back' so characteristic of ankylosing spondylitis. However, good management helps prevent the disease progressing this far. Most people are able to lead very active normal lives.

Exercise and Ankylosing Spondylitis

Exercise is the key to the successful management of ankylosing spondylitis. It is essential to keep the affected joints as mobile as possible. This involves a consistent, active exercise program. Also, you need to be aware of your posture at all times — even when you are sleeping! If the bones are going to fuse together, you want them to be in the most functional position possible.

We have included a selection of exercises specifically for people with ankylosing spondylitis (see page 56). You will also find helpful exercises in the other sections — in particular breathing, neck, hips and other back exercises.

SOFT TISSUE RHEUMATISM — OTHER ACHES AND PAINS

Not all the aches and pains you experience are due to arthritis. With most of them, nature takes its course and they go away of their own accord. We often refer to these rather ill-defined aches and pains as a 'touch of rheumatism'. However, some of them can be categorized.

Fibrositis: This refers to generalized muscular aches and pains, especially in the region of the neck and upper back. Often there are specific points which are very tender to the touch. Fibrositis is often associated with general tension and sleep disturbances. The pain is probably due to increased tension in the muscles. Thus regular exercise and relaxation can be of great help if you suffer from fibrositis.

Neck ache and backache: When we are under stress, we tend to store it in the muscles of our body. The most common areas for holding onto this tension are the neck and lower back. This, combined with poor posture, is one of the main causes of stiffness and aching in the neck and lower back. Again, regular exercise and relaxation can work wonders in relieving the body of tension and encouraging good posture.

Bursitis: In this condition, one or more of the fluid-filled cushions outside the joint become inflamed. Sometimes bursitis is associated with rheumatoid arthritis. Usually, though, it is a localized condition which can occur after an injury, prolonged or repeated pressure, or overuse. The most common sites are the shoulder, the elbow and the knee. The best treatment for bursitis is rest and the use of comfort techniques, but be sure to move the joint through its range of movement a few times each day to prevent stiffness.

Tendonitis and inflammation of muscle attachments: Inflammation of the tendons is known as tendonitis. Common areas for this are on the thumb side of the wrist and at the back of the heel. 'Tennis elbow' (on the outside of the elbow joint) and 'golfers elbow' (on the inside of the elbow joint) are common examples of inflammation of the muscles where they attach to the bone. These problems are usually due to overuse or poor technique. They can be very persistent. You need to avoid whichever activity is aggravating the problem.

Osteoporosis: Osteoporosis is not actually a type of arthritis although it may be associated with arthritis. The bones become weaker and more brittle. As a result, fractures can occur more easily when the bones are put under stress. Women are more commonly affected than men, particularly after menopause.

It is possible to decrease the risk of developing osteoporosis by ensuring that your diet includes plenty of foods rich in calcium, such as milk. Exercise is also important. Regular daily exercise stimulates your bones to grow stronger.

If you do have osteoporosis, be very careful not to put too much stress on your bones by attempting a vigorous exercise program. The exercises described in this book, combined with walking or cycling, are quite suitable.

LET'S FIND OUT ABOUT...

DIET

Some of the most common questions asked by people with arthritis relate to diet: 'Should I eat more of this? Should I avoid these foods? Will it help if I take this supplement?' Often, in magazine articles, people are said to be miraculously cured of their arthritis by following a particular diet. But the answer may not be that simple. There are a number of reasons why it is difficult to determine what caused the person's improvement.

Firstly, don't lose sight of the fact that arthritis is not a single disease, but a name that covers a wide range of very different conditions. This means that what helps one form of arthritis may not work for another.

Secondly, one of the characteristics of arthritis — particularly rheumatoid arthritis — is that it comes and goes. How can we be certain that a particular remission is due to a change of diet?

Also, your weight affects the amount of strain you put on your joints. Most diets, if followed strictly, will result in some loss of weight even if they are not designed to do so.

The final point is that your mental attitude has a great effect on your perception of pain and your ability to cope with it. Enthusiastically embarking on a new diet can be a very positive step towards helping yourself — a move which challenges the influence your arthritis has on you.

All this does not mean that diet is not a significant factor in managing your arthritis. It is. But there are no scientific studies which prove that specific foods are directly related to arthritis. The only exception is gout. People who have had an attack of gout can usually control further episodes by taking certain dietary precautions.

How then can diet help your arthritis? There are two main ways:
- a nutritious well-balanced diet is good for everyone,
- being overweight adds to the problems of arthritic joints.

By eating a nourishing diet, you can be sure that your body is receiving all the necessary nutrients to give you energy, keep you healthy and repair damaged tissues.

People who are overweight put more strain on their joints — especially those of the back and lower limbs. They are generally less active, too, and more prone to other illnesses such as heart and circulatory conditions and diabetes.

The Pyramid Food Plan* is an excellent guide to good nutrition and a balanced diet:

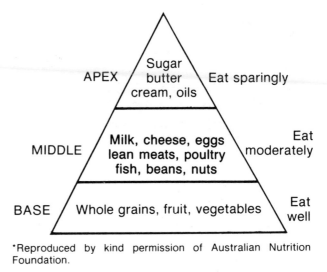

APEX	Sugar butter cream, oils	Eat sparingly
MIDDLE	Milk, cheese, eggs lean meats, poultry fish, beans, nuts	Eat moderately
BASE	Whole grains, fruit, vegetables	Eat well

*Reproduced by kind permission of Australian Nutrition Foundation.

Base: **These foods should form the bulk of your diet. They provide you with energy, supply many nutrients, and have a high fiber content that helps to regulate your bowel func-**

tion. Remember: raw or lightly cooked foods retain more of their nutrients.

Middle: You should eat moderate amounts of foods in this section. They provide the protein so necessary for the maintenance and repair of your body tissues, as well as other nutrients.

Apex: Eat these foods sparingly. Some have a high fat content; others have lots of calories but very little nutritive value.

Try to avoid foods which contain preservatives and other chemical additives. Limit your salt intake, as well as your consumption of alcohol and caffeine. The dangers to your health of cigarette smoking are now well known.

If you are overweight, you need to consume fewer calories than you use up. Exercise and increased activity will certainly help. As far as diet is concerned, concentrate on the lower parts of the pyramid. Don't try to lose too much weight too quickly. Weight that comes off slowly is more likely to stay off.

Some people with rheumatoid arthritis have the problem of being underweight. It's a mistake to try to gain weight by eating sweet rich fatty foods. These supply calories but not a lot of nutriment. Concentrate instead towards the middle of the pyramid, which contains foods that are both nourishing and quite high in calories.

MENTAL ATTITUDE

Your attitude to your arthritis and your expectations about it are two major factors in determining how much effect arthritis has on your life. Anxiety, pain and fatigue are all associated with feelings of depression. It's very easy to let yourself become more and more miserable and less able to cope with your daily activities.

There are many ways to help lift yourself out of this cycle, but the first big step is for you to *decide that you want to help yourself.* Friends and relatives, church and community groups, counsellors, your doctor and other health professionals can all give you guidance, but *you* are the one who is ultimately in control of your own life and your attitude towards it. Once you have a positive focus,

you will probably find that your arthritis no longer bothers you to the same degree.

STRESS

Have you found that your arthritis is worse when you are under physical or emotional stress? This is very common. It seems that when we try to push ourselves too far our bodies start to give way at their weakest links. For people with arthritis, this is their joints.

Sometimes the onset of rheumatoid arthritis coincides with a period of severe stress in a person's life. This is not to say that stress causes arthritis, but it is possibly a contributing factor. And once you have arthritis, it is certainly affected by stress. Medicine today is acknowledging the close relationship between our minds and our bodies.

Of course, it is impossible to rid yourself of all stress in your life. The unexpected can always happen. But you can try to eliminate many unnecessary day-to-day stresses by:
- planning ahead
- being realistic about time and your capabilities
- assessing your priorities
- sharing the responsibilities
- asking for help
- **practicing your relaxation.**

VISITING THE DOCTOR

Aches, pains and minor injuries of our joints are very common. After giving us a few days of discomfort, they usually go away of their own accord. People often wonder whether they should go to their doctor or not. In general, there is not a lot the doctor can do to help these minor non-specific ailments. Probably, you will be advised to rest the part and take some mild form of pain relief.

However, you do not have to suffer in silence in the mistaken belief that 'nothing can be done' or 'doctors don't want to listen'. If you have any one or more of the following symptoms for more than two weeks, then you should make an appointment to see your doctor:

- persistent or recurrent pain in any joint
- swelling in one or more joints
- redness and warmth in a joint
- early morning stiffness
- inability to move a joint normally
- unexplained weight loss, fever or weakness, combined with joint pain.

Once you have gone to your doctor, he or she will take your history and give you a physical examination. This may be all that is needed to establish a diagnosis of arthritis. Sometimes the doctor will want a bit more information in order to confirm the diagnosis or to rule out other possibilities. The most usual investigations are blood tests and x-rays.

Initially, of course, you would start with your local doctor. But if your arthritis is not responding well to treatment or if there is a specific point of concern, you or your doctor may suggest that you see a rheumatologist, a doctor who specializes in rheumatic and arthritic conditions.

However, your main contact will still be with your local doctor, so it is important that you have someone with whom you feel comfortable. Both you and your doctor must have respect for each other. The doctor has the theoretical knowledge and experience of arthritis and its treatment, but you are the only one who knows how your body feels. Find a doctor with whom you can build up a good line of communication, and you are much more likely to get results.

You can help your doctor, too, by preparing the questions you wish to ask and by making sure you understand any advice or instructions given. Don't be embarrassed about asking for further explanations. Your doctor will also be interested in hearing about anything you have found helpful, as your experience can then be passed on to other people. Arthritis is a very individual disease and so needs a personally tailored treatment program. It needs good cooperation between doctor and patient to achieve the most satisfactory results.

MEDICATION

When you first went to a doctor about your arthritis, you were probably given a prescription for some pills or tablets. It's true that medication has a place in the treatment of arthritis, but sometimes both patients and doctors rely too heavily on drugs as the only means of controlling arthritis. All drugs have side-effects, and some people do not tolerate certain drugs as well as others.

When considering drug therapy, it is important to realize the difference between rheumatoid arthritis and osteoarthritis. With rheumatoid arthritis the main problem is inflammation. A reduction of this inflammation will ease the pain. To be effective, medication for the control of inflammation must be ongoing. With osteoarthritis, there is usually no inflammation. The main concern is just pain! Therefore the medication is related to the amount of pain you are experiencing.

There is one important word of caution about drugs. Be sure to consult fully with your doctor about your medication. Don't stop taking a drug or change the dosage without letting your doctor know. Also make sure you understand and follow the dosage instructions. You must remember that you are dealing with potentially damaging substances.

Aspirin: Aspirin is a common drug used for arthritis. It has two main beneficial effects: it relieves pain and it reduces inflammation. Pain relief is obviously important for people with arthritis, but it is aspirin's anti-inflammatory properties which make it (and its related drugs) so useful in dealing with rheumatoid arthritis. The most common side-effect of aspirin is irritation of the lining of the stomach.

Non-steroidal anti-inflammatory drugs: This is a diverse group of drugs which may be classed as aspirin substitutes. Their main action is to reduce inflammation, so they are particularly useful for rheumatoid arthritis. They are derived from different chemical families, so particular drugs are more suited to certain individuals. It may mean a bit of trial and error to discover which is the most suitable drug for your condition. They do not seem to have the same side-effects as aspirin but, because they are newer, we cannot be sure of the hazards of long-term use.

Anti-malarials: The drugs developed for the control of malaria have also been found to help reduce the inflammation of rheumatoid

11

arthritis. They may be used with other drugs and are usually very well tolerated without serious side-effects.

Remittent agents: Everyone has probably heard of gold injections for rheumatoid arthritis. Gold and penicillamine are two different drugs with similar effects on joint inflammation. They can produce a dramatic reduction in symptoms and may even result in a remission. However, they do have potentially hazardous side-effects and must be used with discretion and be carefully monitored.

Cortico-steroids: When it was first developed, cortisone was thought to be a wonder drug for rheumatoid arthritis. Since then, some serious side-effects from long-term use have been found. Cortisone is still useful as a treatment for rheumatoid arthritis, but should be used with great caution and be strictly supervised. Cortisone injections are sometimes given into a particularly troublesome joint. They may give excellent relief lasting for months, but this is not always the case. Although the injections do not have the same side-effects as taking the drug orally, they must still be used discriminately.

Immuno-suppressives: These are very powerful and dangerous drugs which work by suppressing the body's immune system. In all except the most serious forms of arthritis, the risks of side-effects outweigh any potential benefits.

OTHER HEALTH PROFESSIONALS

Part of your treatment program may include physical therapy. A physical therapist knows a lot about how the muscles and joints of your body work. Your physical therapy may include an individualized exercise program, hydrotherapy, heat treatment, appropriate splinting, advice on suitable footwear, instruction on the use of walking aids, education in the best ways to use your body and protect your joints, and information on ways to balance your daily activities.

Occupational therapists are concerned with helping you to function better and more in-

dependently in your daily activities. This may include various aids and devices and suggestions on how to adapt your home so you can do as much as possible for yourself with the least amount of strain on your joints.

Medication is often a cause of concern. Do remember that your local druggist is often a good source of information on how drugs work and can help you understand your doctor's instructions.

SURGERY

There are times when a joint is so badly affected and causes so much pain that the only resort is surgery. You have probably heard or known of people with artificial hips. It is certainly true that these have been a great success in restoring function and relieving the pain of a severely arthritic hip.

Surgery needs to be approached with caution and careful consideration. It is not always a success, although for many people it has given them a new lease on life. If you are thinking of surgery, then it's wise to consult more than one surgeon. Find someone well experienced in the type of operation you require. It is also a good idea to talk to someone who has had the operation you are considering.

Of course, not all arthritic conditions are suitable for surgery. In general, surgery is most useful when the problem is localized to one joint and is most successful for the larger joints such as the hip and knee. Joint replacement has been a great help to people with severe arthritis in the hip or knee. Other joints (shoulder, ankle, elbow, fingers) are being worked on, and are being operated on with greater success.

COMFORT TECHNIQUES

You have probably found that it is the continual day-to-day pain and discomfort of arthritis that is most upsetting. To cope better with this, you can build up a store of techniques which you know will help to make you more comfortable. This is a big part of 'living with arthritis'. These comfort techniques can make quite a difference to the amount of pain relief you require from drugs:

- Usually warmth helps to ease the pain. Wrap a towel around a hot water bottle or a hot pack (available from druggists) and cover the painful area. *Caution: this should feel warm, not hot. Be especially careful if you have sensitive skin.*

- There are many heat rubs available which you can massage into your joints. *Caution: never use these with other forms of direct heat, and be careful if you have sensitive skin.*

- Soak your hands or feet in a basin of warm water or your whole body in a warm bath.

- A gentle soothing massage from friendly hands is very comforting.

- During the day, thermal underwear, gloves and scarves help keep you warm; and when you are considering what to wear, remember that wool retains warmth better than synthetic materials.

- Electric blankets, woollen mattress pads, and feather comforters help keep you warm through the night.

- Try wearing socks, gloves, leg warmers, knee or elbow socks to bed and retain the warmth in your joints.

- If possible, warm the room before you get up.

Do not apply heat to a hot swollen joint — it won't help. If at any time heat is making your joint feel worse instead of more comfortable, then don't keep on with it.

JOINT PROTECTION

If you have arthritis, you need to be constantly aware of how much stress you are putting on your joints. Your aim is to prevent undue strain on your joints, so as to minimize your pain and keep them working for as long as possible. You need to balance activity with rest. Do not use your joints unnecessarily if they are painful — try to avoid using them at all if they are hot and swollen.

Joint protection means using your joints wisely. Make sure that you lift, stand and move in a way that puts least stress on your joints (refer pages 77–9). Use the larger stronger joints to do the work, and try to distribute any load you are carrying over several joints. Think before you try to do a particular task. You are very likely to discover an easier, less stressful way of doing it.

There are various aids and devices which have been developed to take the strain off tender joints. Do you know that you can obtain gadgets which help you to put on stockings and socks, comb your hair, open cans and jars, turn on taps, hold pens and cutlery, pick things up off the floor, do the gardening, pull out plugs from the wall and many other daily activities? An occupational therapist or the Arthritis Foundation (page 81) can give you advice on where to obtain these useful devices.

THE WEATHER

Do you believe you can predict the weather with at least as much accuracy as the Weather Bureau? Many people find that their arthritis seems to be aggravated by an impending change of weather — i.e. when the barometric pressure is rising or falling.

As far as general climate is concerned, it seems that dampness and humidity have the most disturbing effects, so both cold and wet days or hot and humid ones can be very uncomfortable. Windy changeable weather is also not well tolerated. Although the climate does not seem to be related to the prevalence of arthritis, the day-to-day weather often has some bearing on the amount of pain experienced in arthritic joints.

It is worth noting whether the weather seems to affect your arthritis, because it may account for a particularly bad day and at least you know it will pass!

YOUR EXERCISE PROGRAM

WHY EXERCISE?

We have already mentioned some of the ways in which exercise can benefit people with arthritis. This book, then, is about the relationship between *exercise* and *arthritis*.

A regular program of appropriate exercises will:
- keep your joints mobile
- increase your muscle strength
- strengthen your bones and ligaments
- prevent joint deformities
- provide nourishment to your joints
- maintain and increase your ability to perform daily tasks
- **increase your general fitness and sense of well-being.**

TYPES OF EXERCISE

There are many different exercises, but all of them fall into three basic categories: mobility, strengthening and aerobic. Often a particular exercise will contain elements of more than one type. A good general exercise program should incorporate all three types.
1. *Mobility (or stretching) exercises.* These are the exercises which move your joints through their full range of motion. Their purpose is to maintain or increase the amount of movement in a joint. They will help to decrease pain and improve the joint's functional ability.

2. *Strengthening exercises.* The purpose of these exercises is to increase the strength of the muscles which move, support and protect your joints. Muscle wasting and weakness often accompany painful joints, putting even more strain on them. A combination of mobility and strengthening exercises is important because you need to have control of the amount of movement in your joints, as well as giving them as

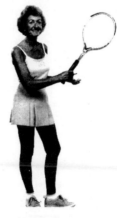

An aerobic exercise

much support as possible.
3. *Aerobic (or endurance) exercises.* These are the more general activities — e.g., walking, swimming, cycling, playing sports, dancing and jogging — which help to increase your overall fitness level. You will stimulate your lungs and cardiovascular system if you exercise large muscle groups for a period of at least 20 minutes. Half an hour of aerobic exercise 2-3 times per week will improve your fitness and enhance your feeling of well-being.

EXERCISE WITH CARE

For your exercise program, you need to choose activities that do not put too much strain on your joints. You can well imagine that weightlifting is not the best exercise for arthritic shoulder, nor is downhill skiing sensible if you have osteoarthritis in your knee. Contact sports are obviously unwise for people with arthritis. Still, do not despair: there are plenty of other sports and activities less likely to cause damage, such as tennis, bowling, golf, folk-dancing and swimming. Use your common sense and choose something that does not put too much stress on your affected joints. And be sure to take it easy when your joints are painful.

If you are doing anything that involves running or walking, be sure to wear good supportive walking or jogging shoes — the kind that will absorb some of the shock and so protect your joints.

Swimming and other water activities are excellent for people with arthritis. The buoyancy of water relieves much of the weight from your joints. Many of the exercises in this book can be done in the water.

At first, it is difficult to know how much exercise to do or when you have done too much. But experience is a great teacher. A good rule to go by is that, if you experience *exercise-induced pain for more than two hours* after the exercise period, then you have overdone it. Next time do a little less. Some muscle soreness is quite normal after unaccustomed exercise. But you want to avoid the pain caused by your joints being irritated by too much exercise.

Pain, as we have said, is a warning you are causing damage to your body. The cliche that 'the more it hurts, the more good it's doing' is simply not true.

The exercises described in this book are all free active movements without assistance or resistance from any outside force. They have been developed for people with mild to moderate arthritis. If you practice them regularly, you will strengthen your muscles and stretch your joints. The exercises won't put excess strain on your joints, although some people will not be able to do all the exercises. *Do not do any exercise which causes you pain*. Do, however, make a gentle attempt at the same exercise a week or so later. There may be a pleasant surprise in store for you. Your stronger muscles and joints may now allow you to do the exercise more easily.

WHO SHOULD EXERCISE

The exercise program described in this book has been developed to suit long-term mild-to-moderate arthritic problems. This means that your arthritis has been around for a while, but you don't have marked joint deformities, and in general your arthritis does not greatly hinder you in your normal daily activities.

The program is still suitable if you have had a hip or knee replacement, provided you take note of the precautions mentioned with particular exercises. It is possible to adapt many of the exercises if you have more severe arthritis, but be sure to consult a physical therapist or your doctor first. If you have any questions about the suitability of a particular exercise, you should seek professional help.

WHAT TO EXERCISE

No doubt you have certain parts of your body giving you more problems than others, and of course the bothersome part may change from time to time. When you start your program concentrate on one or two areas at a time, rather than trying to fix everything at once. You may even be surprised to find that the improvement in one part is reflected throughout the rest of your body.

However, over the course of the week go through all the exercises, even those which use parts of your body that do not have arthritis . . . yet!

There are two very good reasons for doing this. First, some forms of arthritis affect different parts of the body at various times. You can stay one step ahead by regularly exercising *all* your joints. The other point is that all the joints of your body are actually linked together, so that a problem in one part will affect the load placed on the joint next to it and so on through your body. Your joints do not work as isolated units but rather as moving parts of a whole functional body. Exercising

16

all your joints will give support to present problem areas and will help prevent future problems.

WHEN TO EXERCISE

Any time of day will do. Only you can choose the most suitable time. But here are some general guidelines and considerations which may help you:
- you need an uninterrupted 15–30 minutes per day
- choose a time of day when you are feeling near your best — not when you are tired or in pain
- if you are taking medication, try to exercise about half an hour after your regular dose — when it is at its most effective
- don't exercise on a full stomach
- break your exercise session into more than one period, if you wish.

WHERE TO EXERCISE

The room you use needs to be well ventilated and neither too cold nor too warm. Make sure you have enough space in which to stretch out. You don't want to knock over your favorite crystal vase! In warm sunny weather, think about going into the fresh air for your exercise session.

For the floor exercises, you might be more comfortable lying on a mat or piece of foam. If you cannot get down onto the floor, lie on the bed provided it has a firm base, but a bed is not as satisfactory as the floor. For the exercises done sitting, use a firm-based chair or stool that is the right height to support your thighs with your feet flat on the floor.

WHAT TO WEAR

The clothes you wear for exercising should allow you to move freely and keep you warm. Just be careful not to cool off too quickly after your exercise period. Put back on any clothes you removed as you warmed up through your exercise session.

BEFORE YOU EXERCISE

If you are feeling very stiff and sore, you could perhaps spend 15–20 minutes warming your joints with one of the comfort techniques described on page 15. The relief from pain and the extra blood flow in the area will allow you to move more easily. *Do not, however, take extra medication* to mask the pain you might feel during exercises. After all, pain is an indication you might be causing damage.

HOW TO EXERCISE

To get the greatest benefit from exercises, give yourself enough time to do them properly. If your time is limited, it is better to do less exercises well, rather than rushing through a greater number.

When you are performing a particular exercise, concentrate on the part of your body which is being exercised. Feel how your joint is moving and which muscles are working. This awareness will help you to coordinate the movement. Make your movements smooth, rhythmic and at an easy pace. You may overstrain your joints if you try to move too vigorously.

We have suggested that you start with 2–4 repetitions of each exercise. If you have no painful after-effects, gradually build this up to 5–6 at the rate of one extra repetition per week. If the joint becomes tender, then decrease the number of repetitions. Refrain from exercising a joint that has 'flared-up' and become hot, swollen and painful. Just move the joint very gently through its range of movement twice a day.

And don't forget to keep breathing as you exercise! Your muscles need oxygen in order to work. Sometimes you can find yourself holding your breath unintentionally, particularly with difficult or uncomfortable movements. Coordinating movement with your breathing can help you exercise. Breathe in with one part of the movement, then breathe out with another. In general, think of breathing in (expanding your chest) with opening or lifting movements, and breathing out (deflating the chest) with closing movements.

17

Some people find their exercise sessions much more enjoyable if they move to music. This is a good idea, but a word of caution about your choice of music. If it has a strong fast beat, you may be tempted to keep in time and so move your joints too vigorously. Slow gentle background music or pleasant easy-listening music is best.

Beware of the bug of over-enthusiasm. It usually results in the activity being short-lived. If you have not done much exercise recently, a sudden burst of activity is likely to do more harm than good. It can leave you feeling all your good intentions have been wasted. Be sensible. Follow the guidelines, gradually increasing the amount of exercise. It is not true that, if a little bit is good for you, more of it should be better!

Don't be deterred if the benefits of your exercise program are not immediately obvious. Rome was not built in a day, and miracles are very rare! Your arthritis has probably been developing over many years, so it is unreasonable to expect it to improve overnight. It is more likely that you will barely notice the subtle improvements until you suddenly realize you are doing something you could not do before. For the first week or two, despite all precautions, your general pain level may increase as your joints and muscles move in unaccustomed ways. If you continue doing the exercises regularly and carefully, this should soon pass. If it doesn't, or if the pain is severe, then stop and see your doctor.

Your exercise session can become an enjoyable part of your daily routine. There will, of course, be times when you feel as though you can't be bothered or you haven't got time. Once you start putting things off, it's harder to begin the routine again. We hope the variety of exercises presented in this book and the benefits you get from doing them will stimulate you to keep going.

AFTER YOU EXERCISE

The time following an exercise period is an ideal time to practice relaxation. Muscles and joints are then ready to release their tension. If you do not have time for a relaxation session, then just allow yourself to ease gradually back into your daily activities. Even though the exercises did not seem so energetic at the time, you could find that you are quite tired afterwards.

Also, be aware of your pain level after your exercise session. You have done too much if you have exercise-induced pain for more than two hours.

COMPLETING YOUR EXERCISE PROGRAM

We have not included any specific aerobic exercises, but these do have an important role in your exercise program. Do some regular activity which exercises your lungs and heart for at least half an hour, two to three times each week. Choose something that you enjoy doing. Swimming, walking and cycling are all excellent aerobic activities which do not overstrain your joints. Remember that if you go for a walk or run, then you also have to come back to your starting point. If you wait until you are weary before returning, you will end up exhausted! For any activity that is new to you, be sure to build it up gradually.

PLANNING YOUR EXERCISE PROGRAM

The exercises in this book have been divided into sections:

Each section includes a short introduction before describing the exercises. This gives some background into what you might expect of arthritis in that area, the purpose of the exercises, and any precautions you need to take.

When you do an exercise for the first time, read through all the instructions before you start to move. Study the pictures and the captions so that you understand the exercise properly.

The Key Exercises have been chosen as the ones which are generally the most important for that body part. Through your own experience or following the advice of your physical therapist or doctor, you may choose your own Key Exercises. Key Exercises are marked by a star (★).

You are now able to develop your own individual exercise program. The suggested daily routine would include:

In order to fit in all the exercises over the week, add one extra body part to your exercise period each day, or include two or three longer sessions during the week.

The following chart will help you to keep track of your weekly exercise program. Each day you can tick off what you have done and add any comments. An example of Monday's and Tuesday's programs has been given, assuming the hip to be the main problem.

Morning Wake Up	If you have early morning stiffness

Warm Up
All exercises for your
  main problem areas
Key Exercises for the
  rest of your body
Cool Down
	During the day

	Monday	Tuesday	Wednesday	Thursday	Friday	Saturday	Sunday
Morning Wake Up	✔	✔					
Warm Up	✔	✔					
Neck	✔ 3 times each						
Arms		✔ 3 times each					
Hands		✔ 3 times each					
Back							
Hips	✔ Ex. 4, 6 painful. 3 times each	✔ Ex. 4, 6 not done. 2 times each					
Knees							
Feet							
Cool Down	✔	✔					
Relaxation	✔ ½ hour						
Amount of pain afterwards	Left hip painful all day.						

Points to remember:

- Try to exercise every day.

- Start with 2–4 of each exercise and gradually build up to 5–6.

- Concentrate on the part you are moving.

- Keep breathing.

- Do not exercise a hot tender joint.

- Do not do any exercise which causes severe pain.

- Take note of relevant precautions.

- Read the instructions properly.

- You have done too much if you experience exercise-induced pain for more than two hours.

- **Consult a physical therapist or doctor if you are doubtful about an exercise.**

- Enjoy yourself.

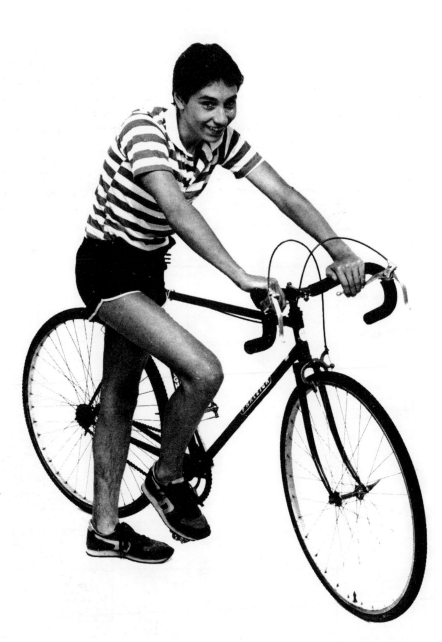

MORNING WAKE UP

Do you find that your joints are stiff and difficult to move when you wake up in the morning? This is a common problem, particularly for people with rheumatoid arthritis.

Morning Wake Up is a sequence of exercises which move all the main joints of your body. This will help to get you moving and out of bed in the morning.

How you feel when you wake up often depends on how well you slept and rested during the night. A good night's sleep is really important. It's much harder to cope with aches and pains if you are tired.

You should give your body the best support possible with a good firm mattress. A low pillow is preferable, especially if you have neck problems. A light down-filled comforter provides as much warmth as three or four blankets,. and eases the weight on your body through the night. It's also a lot easier to make the bed!

A bed that has been nicely warmed up by an electric blanket is comforting to climb into. Also, a good woollen mattress pad provides a bit of a cushion to your body and helps to keep in the warmth.

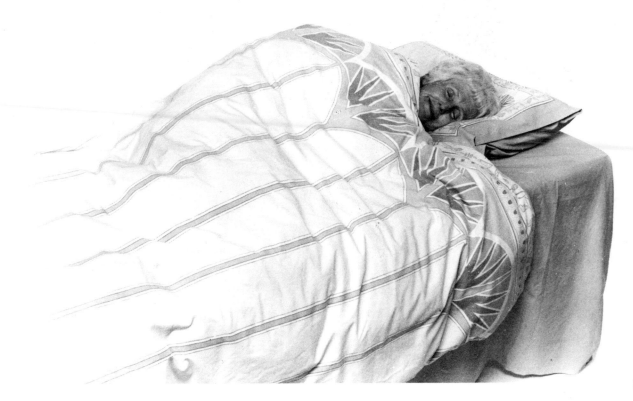

Getting to sleep or waking up during the night can be a worry. There are no easy solutions, but we have included a few suggestions to help you relax and fall asleep (page 75). Give them a try.

However, even after a really good night's sleep, you may still wake up feeling that you can't move. This is when you need Morning Wake Up to help get yourself up and about.

Make sure you give yourself about 10–15 minutes to go slowly through the whole sequence. You must gently encourage your joints to move, not force them. Do each of the movements two or three times, maybe an extra couple of times for your stiffest joints. You can include exercises from other parts of the book if you think they would be particularly helpful. If you are running short of time in the morning, just do the breathing (Exercise 1), then choose the exercises which move your problem joints.

Getting out of bed is easier when you use the method shown in Exercise 10. In this way, you use the body's own momentum, which puts less strain on your joints.

We have left the covers off the model so that you can see what she is doing. However, it is important for you to keep warm, so don't follow her example. Keep under the covers. Just make sure they are loose enough so that you can move easily.

Have a good morning!

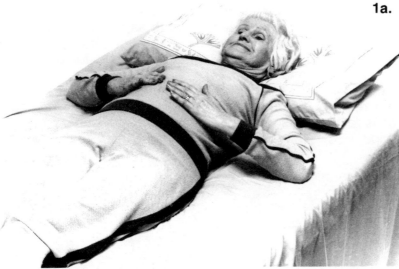

1a.

1. Start: Lie with hands on your lower ribs.

1a. Breathe in slowly and easily. Feel your chest expand under your hands. Let your breath 'sigh' out.

1b. Open your mouth wide and yawn.

1c. Breathe in, then gently blow the air out. Continue blowing out until your lungs are empty; let yourself breathe in.

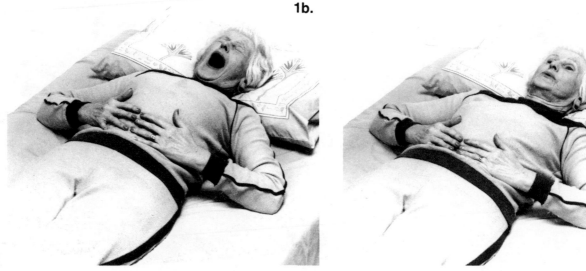

1b.

1c.

2. Start: Lie with your legs straight.

2a. Bend back your toes.

2b. Gently curl your toes under.

2c. Bend back your foot.

2d. Push your foot down.

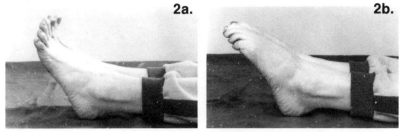
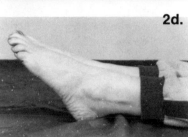
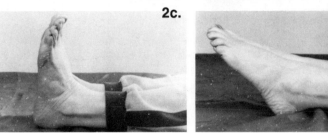

3. Start: Lie with your legs straight.

Slide your heel up towards your bottom. Straighten your leg out along the bed. Repeat with the other leg.

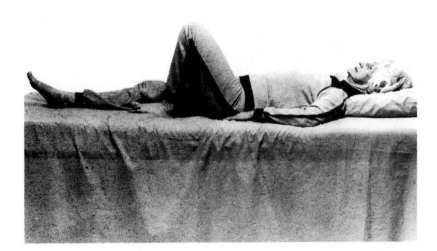

4. Start: Lie with both knees bent.

4a. Gently arch your back.

4b. Flatten your back onto the bed and tilt your pelvis upwards by tightening your buttocks and stomach muscles.

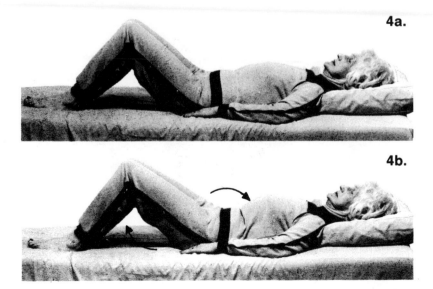

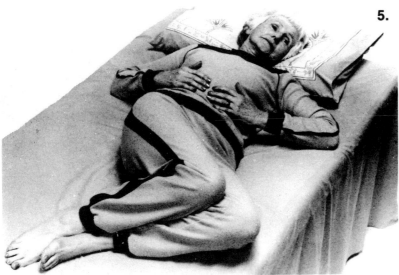

5.

5. Start: Lie with both knees bent.

Gently roll your knees from side to side.

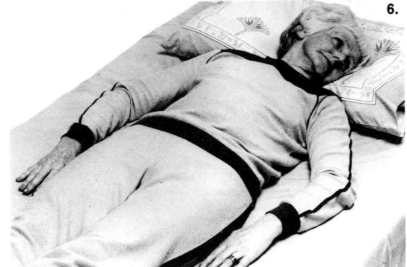

6.

6. Start: Lie looking upwards.

Gently roll your head from side to side.

7. Start: Lie with your arms by your sides.

7a. Gently roll your arms outwards, turning your palms up.

7b. Gently roll your arms inwards, turning your palms down.

7a.

7b.

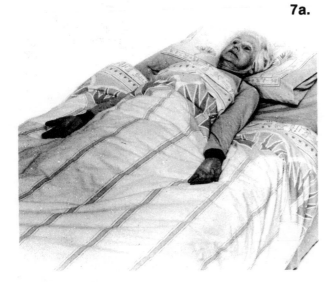 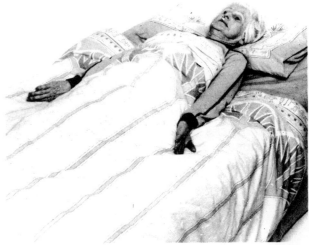

8. Start: Lie with your arms by your sides.

8a. Stretch out your fingers.

8b. Gently curl your fingers into your palm.

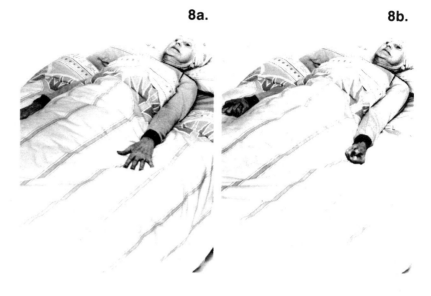

8a. **8b.**

9. Start: Lie with your hands by your sides on top of the covers.

9a. Gently curl up your fingers and bring your fists to your shoulders.

9b. Stretch your arms upwards, opening out your fingers.

9c. Lower your elbows to the bed and touch your shoulders with your fingertips.

9d. Straighten your arms down by your sides.

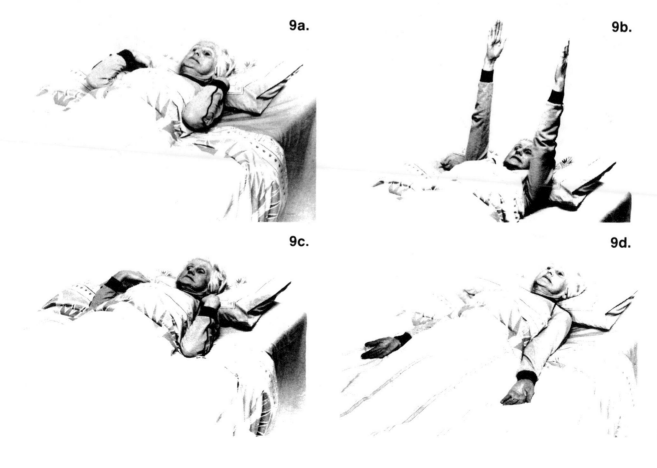

9a. **9b.**

9c. **9d.**

GETTING OUT OF BED

10. Start: Lie with both knees bent up. Use a continuous flowing movement.

10a. Roll to one side, stretching across your body with the top arm.

10b–d. Pivot on your bottom so your legs swing down over the edge of the bed and your body swings upward. Assist the movement, pushing with your top hand and bottom elbow.

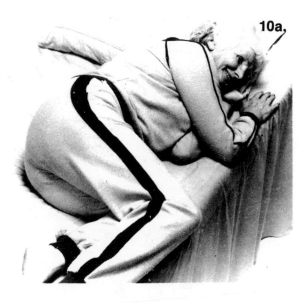

10a.

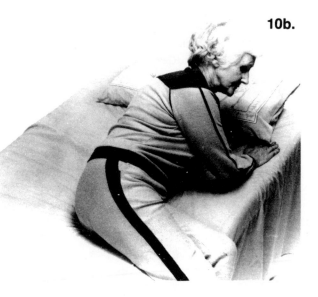

10b.

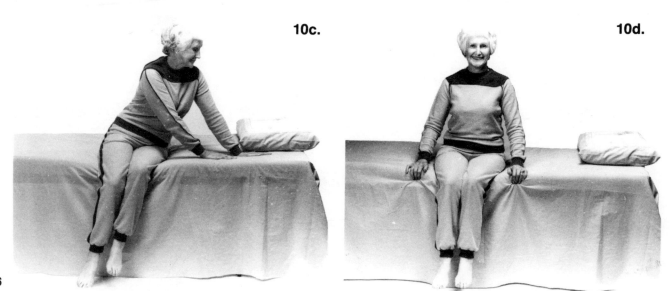

10c.

10d.

WARM UP

It is a good idea to warm up your whole body before you start doing exercises for your specific problem areas — particularly if you have been sitting still for a while. Arthritic joints can stiffen up very easily. Warming up may also include some of the pre-exercise techniques discussed on page 13.

This Warm Up sequence is a gentle way of starting to move. It helps to get both you and your joints into the mood for exercise. Once your muscles start working, your circulation increases. It is the blood which transports oxygen, energy and nourishment to your body and takes away the waste products. As the circulation to your joints and muscles increases, they warm up and are able to move more easily. This means you can gradually work up to more difficult exercises after starting with some easy movements.

As we have said, your whole body needs exercise, not just those joints that are giving you trouble. Remember, regular exercise will help prevent further problems. If you are very short of time one day, just doing the Warm Up will ensure you have moved all the main joints of your body.

You can do the Warm Up either sitting on a chair or standing up. It depends which you find most comfortable.

Exercises 1–6 can all be done sitting or standing. If you want to remain sitting, finish with Exercises 7 and 8. If you don't mind weight bearing, then add Exercises 9 and 10.

Do each exercise 2–4 times.

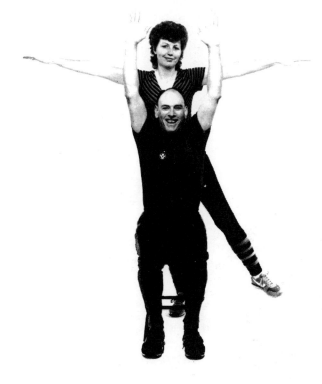

27

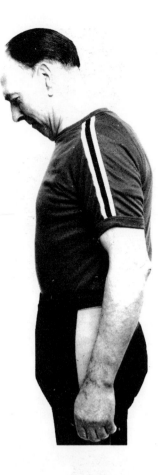

1.

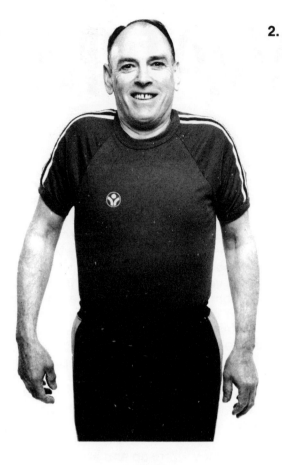

2.

Start your Warm Up with five slow full breaths. Let each breath 'sigh' out.

1. Start: Breathe in.

Breath *out* as you bend your head forward. Breathe *in* as you lift your head up. *Do not bend your head backwards.*

2. Start: Look straight ahead.

Breathe *in* as you lift up your shoulders. Breathe *out* as you relax your shoulders.

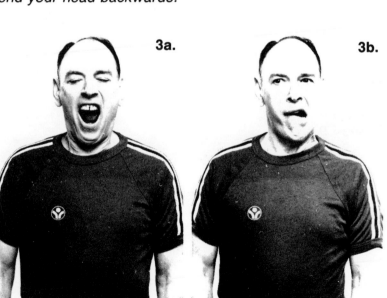

3a.

3b.

3. Start: With your mouth closed.

3a. Stretch your mouth open and let yourself 'yawn'.

3b. Imagine you are chewing a large piece of sticky toffee. Stretch your mouth in all directions for 5–10 seconds.

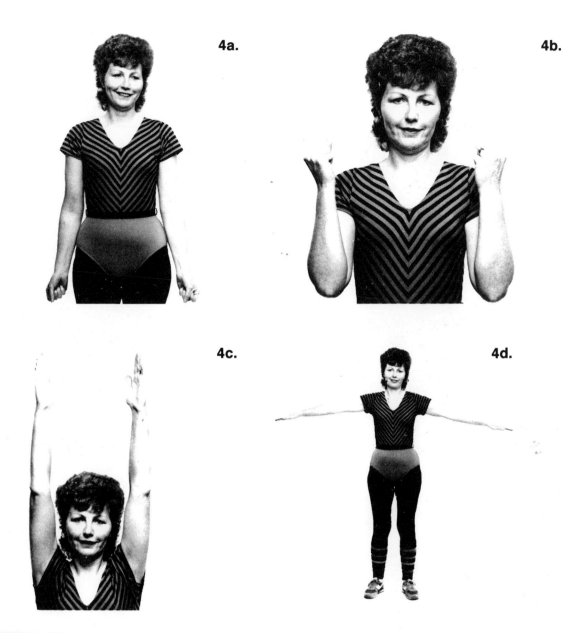

4a.

4b.

4c.

4d.

4. Start: Sit or stand with your arms by your sides.

4a. Curl your fingers into a loose fist.

4b. Bring your hands up to your shoulders.

4c. Spread open your fingers as you stretch your arms upwards, with your palms facing each other.

4d. Lower your arms sideways, with your palms facing downwards.

5a.

5b.

6.

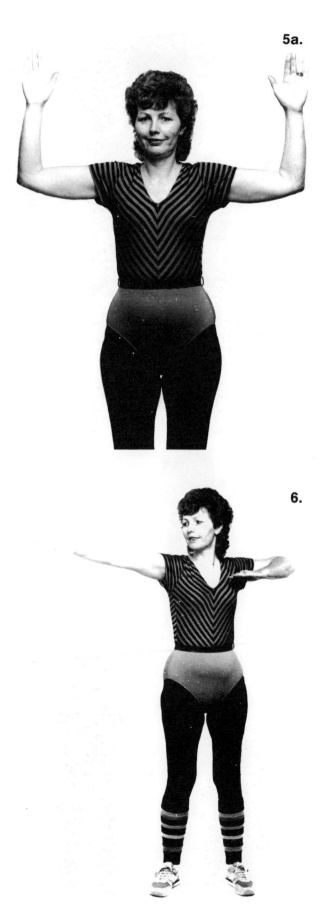

5. Start: Sit or stand with your arms held out to the sides, elbows at right angles and palms facing forwards. Keep your elbows at shoulder level.

5a. Breathe *in* as you stretch backwards with your arms.

5b. Breathe *out* as you bring your elbows and palms together.

6. Start: Sit or stand, looking straight ahead.

Stretch forward with one arm and backward with the other elbow. Let yourself twist at the waist. Look at your front hand. Change arms and twist the other way.

7. Start: Sit with both feet flat on the floor.

Lift the heel of each foot alternately.

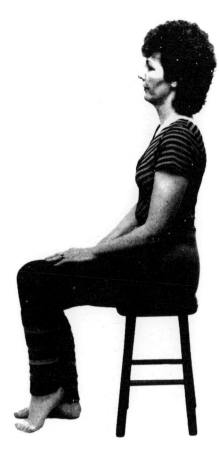

7.

8. Start: Sit up straight with both feet flat on the floor.

Keep your feet on the floor and your back straight. Rock your body around in a circle.

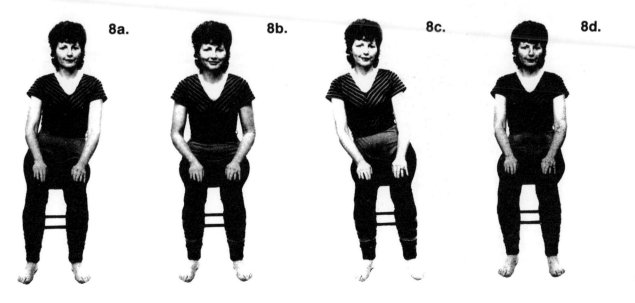

8a.

8b.

8c.

8d.

9a.

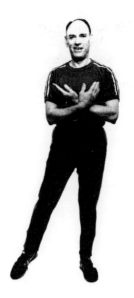

9b.

9. Start: Stand with feet apart.

9a. Breathe *in* as you rock your weight over onto one leg and lift your arms out sideways.

9b. Breathe *out* as you rock over onto the other leg and swing your arms down and across your body.

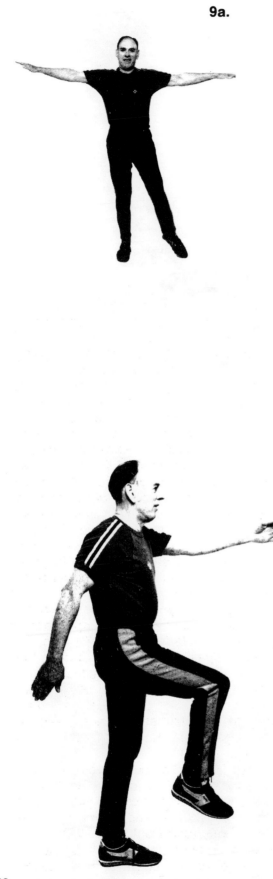

10. Start: Stand with your feet together and arms by your sides.

Mark time by stretching one arm forward and the other arm backward. Lift the opposite knee to the forward arm. Change arms and legs.

NECK

You might well call someone who keeps bothering you a 'pain in the neck'. This common usage suggests just how troublesome neck pain can be.

The neck is the upper part of the spine and is made up of seven bones, or vertebrae, stacked one on top of each other. They all work together to allow your head to move in many directions.

Pain in the neck can be caused by various things — one of which is arthritis. Actual arthritis in the neck means that the joints between the vertebrae have been affected.

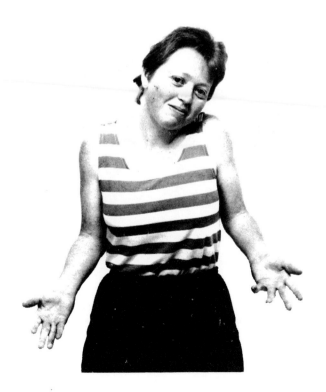

Arthritis in the neck is often associated with one-sided headaches or pain, numbness and tingling down one arm. This is called 'referred pain'. It is due to irritation of the nerves going up to your head or down your arm.

The neck has a large range of movement. This means that we can easily watch what is going on around us. You have probably found that life is more difficult with a stiff neck! However, greater mobility means a sacrifice in stability. So the muscles and ligaments that support the neck are easily strained and over-stretched. For instance, this is what happens when you twist your neck or sleep in an unusual position. Also, in a whiplash injury the head is swung uncontrollably forward and backward. The joints are forced way beyond their normal limits, which causes damage to the supporting soft tissues of the neck.

We often carry a lot of general tension in the muscles around the neck and upper back, making a neck problem worse. If the muscles are tense or in spasm, they tend to squash the joints of the neck together, causing more pain. Of course, pain in the neck can also lead to increased tension in the muscles, thus creating a cycle of pain and tension. Tension in the muscles of the head and neck often result in a headache.

Your head is quite heavy. It weighs about 10 lbs.! A lot of effort is needed to hold it upright. You will put less strain on your neck if you keep it lengthened and in line with the rest of your body (see Posture, p. 77).

Avoid any movement which tends to squash the vertebrae together. This means any exercise which makes your head bend backwards. Also, be aware of how you hold your head. Do you have your chin poking forward? This position puts the same stress on the joints of your neck as bending your head backwards. Imagine that the *crown* of your head is attached to a balloon, and let your head float like the balloon. But don't try too hard to hold your head in the correct position. This will only increase the strain. Exercise 2 will help to improve the way you balance your head on your neck.

You may wonder why we have included eye exercises in the neck section. The reason is that you can take some of the strain off a sore and stiff neck by making your eyes do some of the work for you.

A final word of caution: the neck is a delicate part of the body, so be careful with these exercises. If any of them causes markedly increased neck pain or pain, numbness or tingling radiating down your arm, then don't do them.

Start with 2–4 of each exercise.

The key exercises for this section are 2, 3, 4, 5 and 6.

1. Start: Look straight ahead. Keep your head still throughout.

1a, b. Move only your eyes and look from side to side.

1c, d. Move only your eyes and look up and down.

1a.   **1b.**   **1c.**   **1d.**

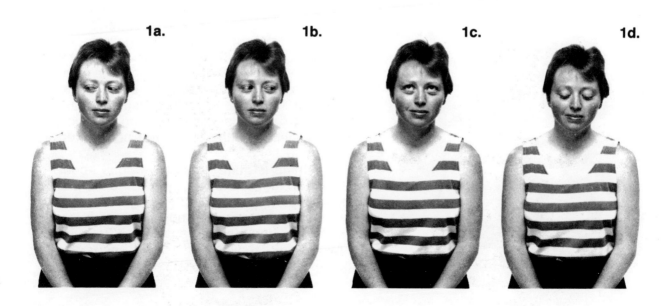

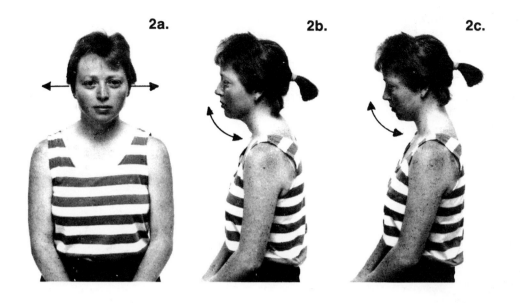

2a. **2b.** **2c.**

★ **2a. Start:** Imagine you have a horizontal line (axis) going through your head, just behind your earlobes.

2b, c. Nod your head up and down around this axis without moving your neck. Finish with your chin slightly dropped.

★ **3. Start:** Look straight ahead with your chin slightly dropped.

Bend your head forward, keeping your chin tucked in. Straighten up but *do not bend your head backwards.*

★ **4. Start:** Look straight ahead, with your chin slightly dropped.

Turn your head and look over alternate shoulders.

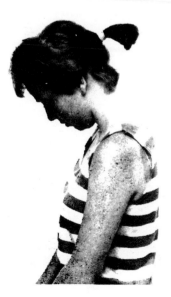

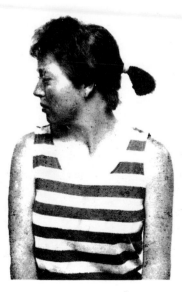

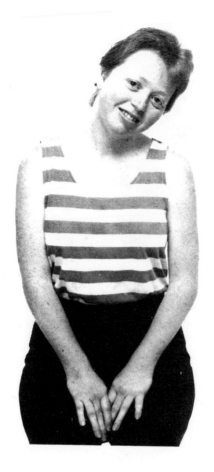

★ **5. Start:** Look straight ahead with your chin slightly dropped.

Keep looking straight ahead and bend your head sideways, taking your ear towards your shoulder. *Do not* lift your shoulder. Bend your head to the other side.

★ **6. Start:** Look straight ahead with your shoulders relaxed.

6a–d. Roll your shoulders in a circular movement — forwards, up, backwards and down.

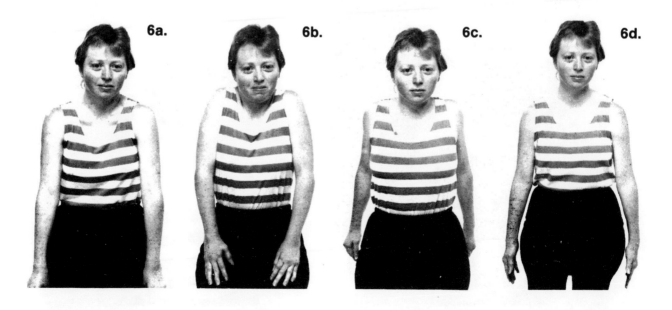

6a. **6b.** **6c.** **6d.**

ARMS

Here are some exercises for your shoulders and elbows. These joints are more usually affected by rheumatoid arthritis than osteoarthritis. They are also common sites for bursitis and tendonitis.

The shoulder is the most flexible joint in your body. Normally it is able to perform many complex movements. If there is any injury to a shoulder joint, it may try to protect itself from further hurt by becoming 'frozen'.

A frozen shoulder can become permanently stiff if it is not exercised properly. Concentrate on Exercises 1–2 if the amount of movement in your shoulder is very limited. These are gentle exercises that will gradually help to increase your shoulder mobility. If your shoulders are reasonably mobile, don't bother with these. Start with Exercise 3.

It doesn't matter whether you sit or stand to do these arm exercises — whichever you find more comfortable.

Start with 2–4 repetitions of each exercise.

The key arm exercises are 4, 5 and 6.

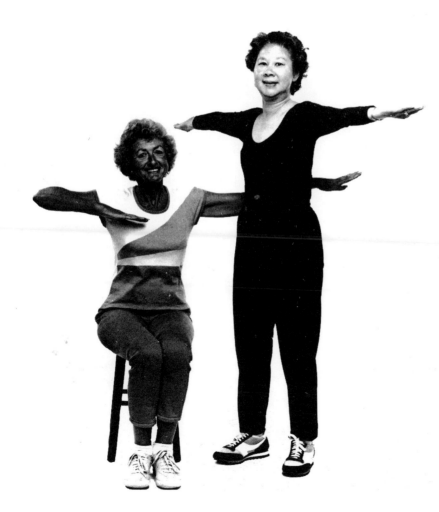

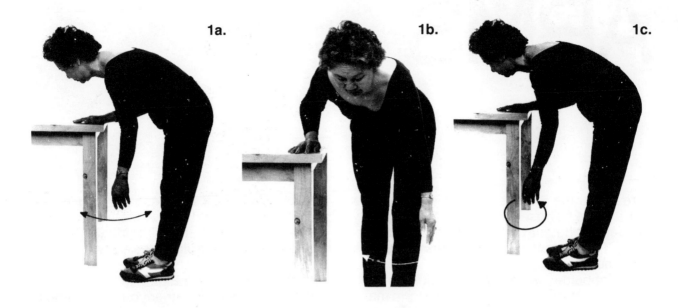

1a.   **1b.**   **1c.**

1. Start: Lean forward on one elbow, onto a table or the back of a chair. Let the other arm hang down. Let the weight of your arm do the swinging like a pendulum; do not let the movement get out of control.

1a. Swing your arm gently forward and back, like a pendulum.

1b. Swing your arm gently out and across your body, like a pendulum.

1c. Swing your arm around in small circles. Reverse direction.

2. Start: Stand about half an arm's length away from a wall.

2a. Face the wall. Walk your fingers upwards as far as you can.

2b. Stand with your side to the wall. Walk your fingers up as far as you can.

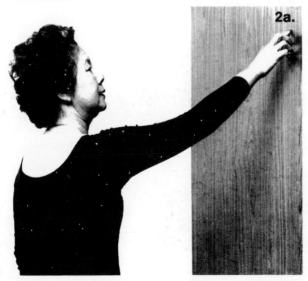

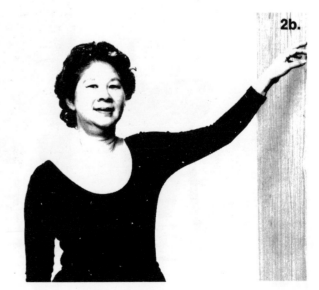

3. Start: Sit or stand with your arms by your sides.

3a. Lift both arms out sideways to shoulder level, palms facing downwards.

3b. Keep your arms at shoulder level. Bend one elbow and touch your shoulder.

3c. Straighten this arm and bend the other elbow.

3d. Straighten out both arms, then lower them slowly to your sides.

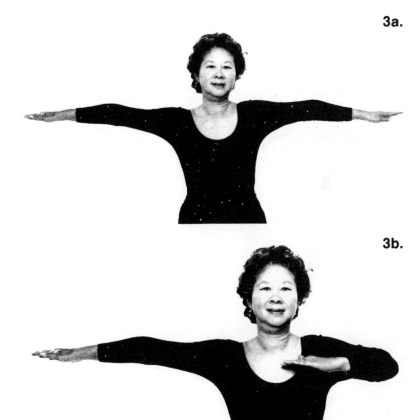

3a.

3b.

3c.

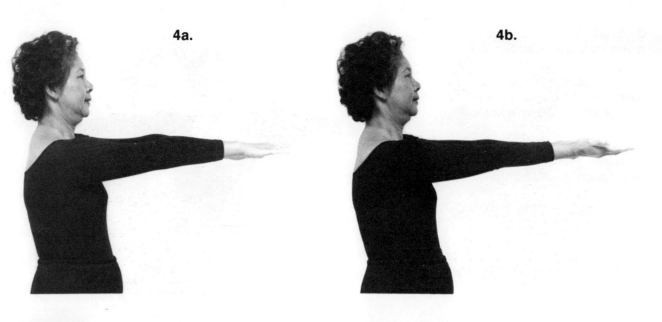

4a.

4b.

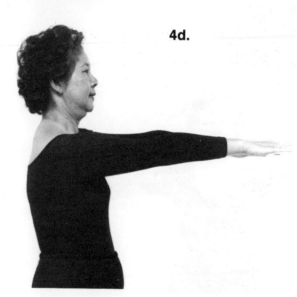

4c.

★ **4. Start:** Sit or stand with your arms by your sides, palms facing backwards.

4a. Lift both arms forward to shoulder level, palms facing down.

4b. Turn your palms up.

4c. Touch your fingertips to your shoulders, letting your elbows drop.

4d. Stretch both arms forward at shoulder level, turning your palms down.

4e. Lower your arms slowly and stretch behind your back. Try to touch your palms together.

4d.

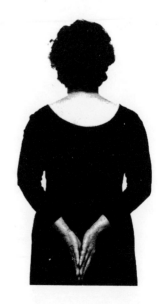

4e.

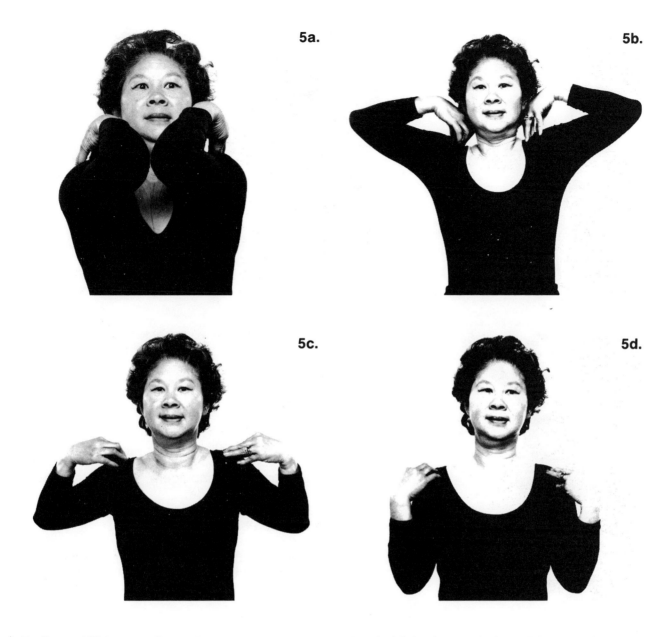

5a.

5b.

5c.

5d.

★ **5. Start:** With your fingertips touching your shoulders.

5a–d. Make large circles with your elbows, bringing them forward, up, back and down. *Breathe in* as you open up and back; *breathe out* as you close down and forward.

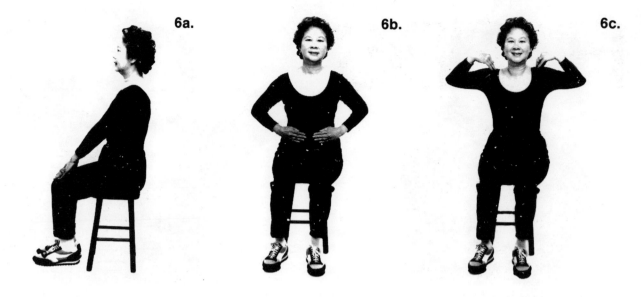

6a.　**6b.**　**6c.**

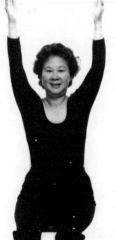

6d.

★ **6. Start:** Sit with your back straight and your feet flat.

6a. Stretch your hands down to touch your knees.

6b. Touch your stomach, keeping your elbows out to the side.

6c. Touch your shoulders, with your elbows lifted out to the side.

6d. Touch behind your head.

6e. Stretch both arms upwards, palms facing each other. Lower your arms with the reverse movements.

6e.

42

HANDS

We use our hands for so many activities that any pain or limitation of movement is soon noticed. Hands are made up of two basic parts with somewhat different functions — the wrist and the fingers.

The main purpose of the wrist is to provide a stable platform from which the much more delicate and mobile fingers can operate. The strength of your hands and fingers is influenced by the position of your wrist. Notice how your wrist bends backwards as you make a fist. A stiff wrist can affect the function of your whole hand.

The large number of finger joints give the fingers their mobility and manipulative ability. They can also compensate for each other to some extent. This means that your hands can still be quite functional even though you have a few stiff joints.

Osteoarthritis usually affects the end joints of the fingers, and you may develop knobby swellings over these joints. They may not look very good but they are not usually very troublesome.

Rheumatoid arthritis in the hands, however, may cause more severe problems. But don't panic — these don't necessarily occur! The joints of the hands most commonly affected by rheumatoid arthritis are the wrists, the knuckles and the middle joints of the fingers. Sometimes the disease process can cause so much damage to the delicate tendons and ligaments that they no longer support the joint in the correct position. Hand deformities can then develop. The most common of these, called 'ulnar deviation', occurs when the hands and fingers start to bend or 'deviate' away from the thumb. If this is happening to your hands, be sure to concentrate on Exercise 8.

If you are having lots of problems with your fingers, exercise each hand separately. Use your other hand to gently assist the movement. But *be careful* not to force your fingers. Your hands are very delicate and need to be coaxed gently into action.

Start with 2–4 of each exercise.
Key exercises: 1, 4, 6.

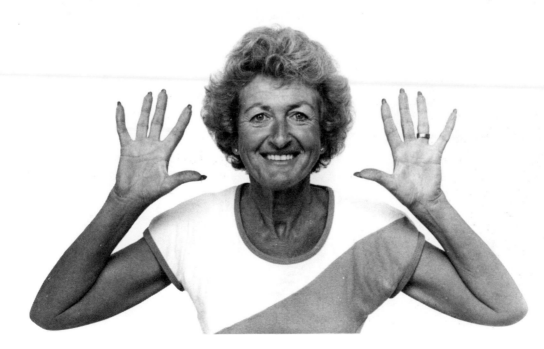

1a.

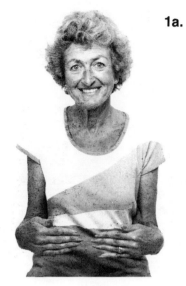

1b.

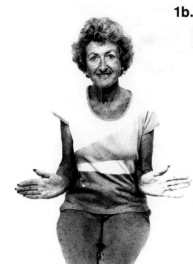

★1. Start: With your elbows tucked in and your palms facing each other.

1a. Bend your wrists forward, bringing your fingers towards each other.

1b. Bend your wrists back so that your palms face the front.

2a. **2b.** **2c.**

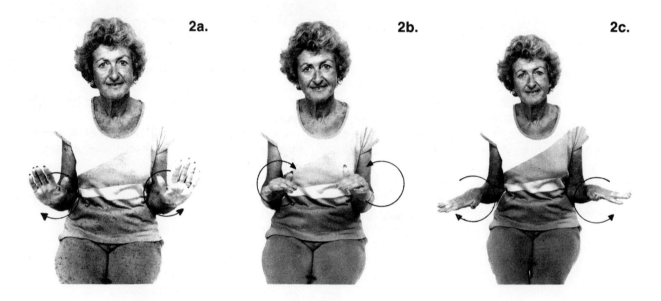

3.

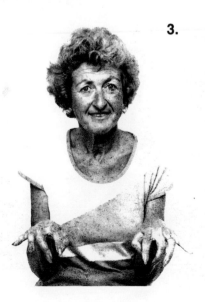

2. Start: With your elbows tucked in.

2a–c. Circle your hands inwards from the wrist — up, in, down and out.

3. Between exercises: relax your fingers by 'playing the piano' with your fingers and thumb.

★ **4. Start:** With your hands in front of you, looking at your palms.

4a. Stretch your thumb across your palm and *gently* close your fingers over it.

4b. Stretch open your fingers and thumb.

4c. *Gently* fold your fingers into your palm and close your thumb over them. *Do not make a tight fist.*

Stretch open your fingers and thumb again.

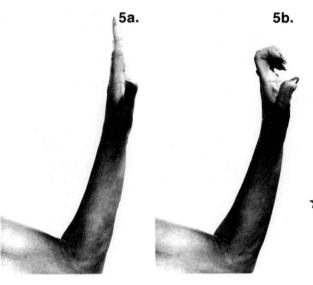

5. Start: With your hands in front of you, palms facing each other.

5a. Straighten out your fingers and thumb.

5b. Bend the top two joints of your fingers down towards the top of your palms. Keep the knuckle joint straight. If your fingers are very stiff, bend each finger individually, helping with the other hand.

★ **6. Start:** Do each hand individually.

6a–d. Touch the tip of your thumb to the tip of each finger in turn. Make the circle as round as you can. Straighten your fingers in between touching each finger.

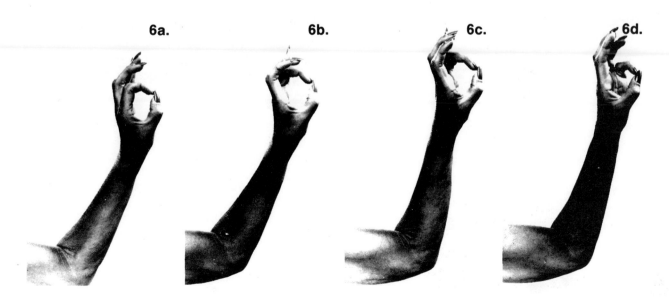

45

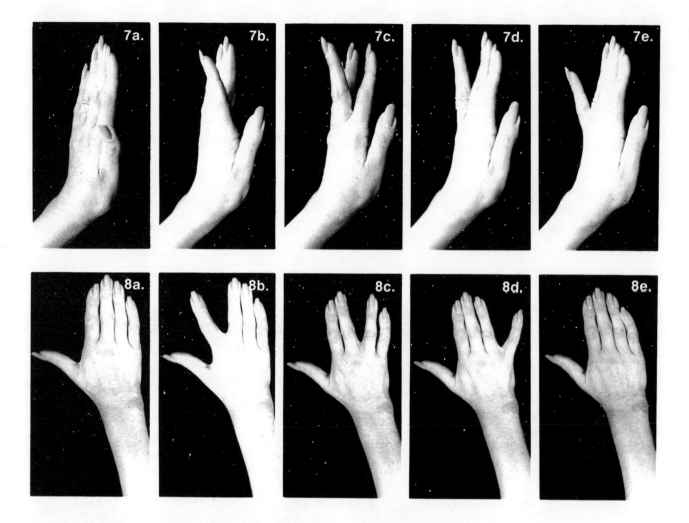

7. Start: Place your hands on a table with your palms down.

7a. Lift your thumb up off the table, then replace it.

7b–e. Lift each finger up off the table, one at a time.

8. Start: Place your hands on a table with your palms down.

8a. Stretch your thumb away from your fingers.

8b–e. Move each finger individually towards your thumb.

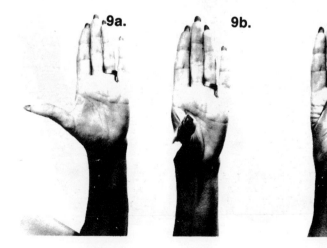

9. Start: Look at the palms of your hands.

9a. Stretch your thumb out sideways away from your palm.

9b. Stretch your thumb forward away from your palm.

9c. Stretch your thumb across your palm to touch the base of your little finger.

BACK

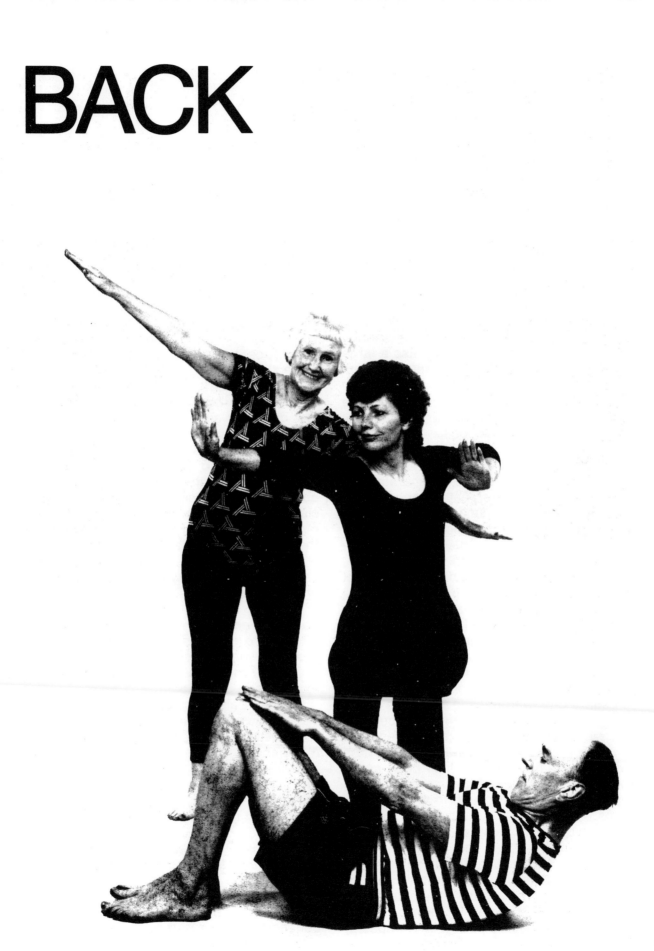

Your back is the central support for your whole body, and as such it must be both strong and flexible. This dual function is achieved by the column of 33 separate bones (called vertebrae) stacked one on top of the other. Each vertebra is separated from its neighbor, above and below, by a spongy shock-absorbing disc. There are also a large number of strong ligaments and muscles supporting your spine.

Straining your back means that you have probably damaged a ligament or muscle. Usually this does not pose much of a long-term problem. A more serious back complaint is what is commonly called a 'slipped disc'. This is not a very accurate term since the disc has not actually slipped out of place. Rather, what has happened is that some of the jelly-like substance inside the disc has been squeezed out. This can irritate one of the nerves going down to your leg.

If you have pain radiating down the back of your leg or any numbness, tingling or muscle weakness in your leg, you have probably been told you have 'sciatica'. All this means is that the sciatic nerve which runs down from your lower back, across your buttock and down the back of your leg is being irritated. It may be because of a slipped disc, but in older people it's usually due to arthritis in the joints of the lower back. As we get older the discs become a bit squashed, so the spaces between the vertebrae are narrower. Osteoarthritis in the lower back may result in small bony spurs growing on the edges of the vertebrae. Both these conditions can cause irritation to the nerves.

When your back is in an acute stage of injury or inflammation, the muscles of the back may go into spasm. This is your back's way of protecting you from further pain or injury. However, the muscle spasm itself can be quite painful resulting in further muscle tension. If your back muscles are in spasm, then you should rest your back and only do very gentle exercises. Remember that your muscles are trying to protect you.

If your back problem is more chronic or if you want to prevent another injury, regular exercise to build up the muscles supporting your back is essential. You have to take good care of your back too! This means maintaining good posture (refer page 77) and lifting correctly (refer page 79).

Two main sets of muscle support your back — *your back muscles*, which you can feel on either side of your spine and, would you believe, *your abdominal muscles!* Abdominal muscles are particularly important in maintaining good posture and in preventing 'swayback'. For chronic low back pain, probably the best exercise is the pelvic tilt (Exercises 6–8). This exercise can be done in various positions. Try all the variations or choose the one you find most comfortable.

If you have osteoporosis of the spine, take care with exercises which bend you forward or sideways (Exercises 2, 3, 5).

We have included some back exercises to be done on hands and knees (Exercises 16–21). *Do not* do these exercises if you have problems with your shoulders, wrists or knees — all the movements are covered in other exercises.

We have also included a section of exercises specifically for people with ankylosing spondylitis (Exercises 18–21). These include a number designed to arch your spine backwards, since ankylosing spondylitis tends to bend you forward. Anyone can do these exercises but *be very careful*. Stop doing them if you experience increased back pain.

Start with 2–4 of each exercise. Cut down or eliminate any exercise which you feel increases your back pain or causes pain going down your leg. After a while you will be able to decide which of these exercises are most beneficial for your particular back problem.

Key exercises: 1, 3, 4, 6, 7, 8, 11.

1.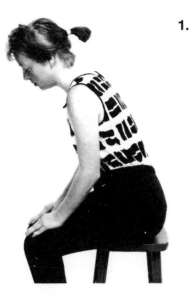

2.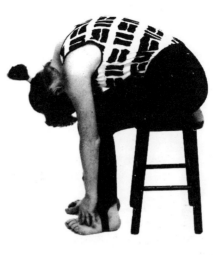

3.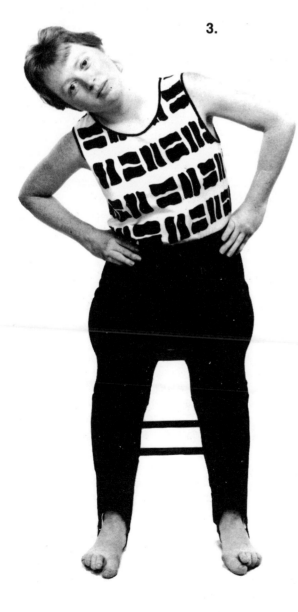

★ **1. Start:** Sit with your feet flat.

Caution: Do this exercise very carefully if you have a hip replacement.

Keep our back and neck in a straight line. Rock forward and then upright as though you are 'hinged' at the hips.

2. Start: Sit with your feet flat.

Caution: Do not do this exercise if you have a hip replacement. Take care if you have osteoporosis of the spine or neck.

Bend your head forward, then slowly curl your body forward, taking your forehead towards your knees. Slowly uncurl from the bottom of your spine until you are sitting upright. Relax your shoulders.

★ **3. Start:** Sit with your feet flat and your hands on your waist.

Caution: Take care if you have osteoporosis of the spine.

Keep looking straight ahead and bend your trunk to one side, over your hand. Straighten up and bend to the other side.

49

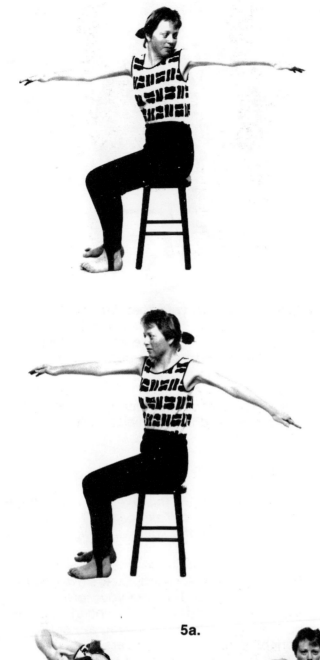

★ **4. Start:** Sit with your feet flat and your arms held out to the side.

4a. Turn your head to look at one hand. Keep looking at your hand as you take your arm backwards, twisting from the waist. Return to face forward, then twist to the other side.

4b. Keep looking straight ahead as you take one arm backwards, twisting from the waist. Return to the front, then take your other arm back.

5. Start: Sit with your feet apart and your fingertips on your shoulders.

Caution: Do not do this exercise if you have a hip replacement. Take care if you have osteoporosis of the spine.

5a. Take one elbow across and down to touch the opposite knee.

5b. Straighten up and gently stretch both elbows backwards. Repeat to the other side.

5a.   **5b.**

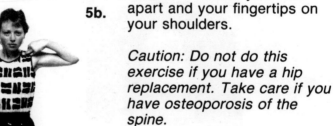

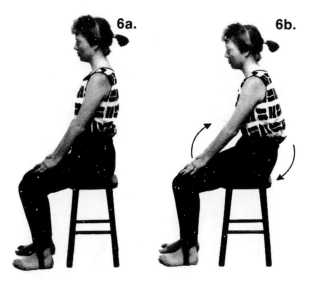
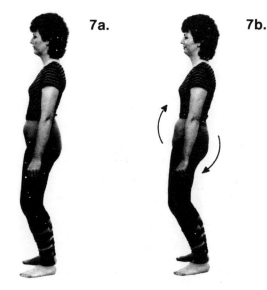

Pelvic rock: The movement is one of 'rocking' your pelvis backward and forward. Do not move your upper body.

★ **6. Start:** Sit up straight with your feet on the floor.

6a. *Gently* arch your lower back. (Rock your pelvis backward.)

6b. Tuck your pelvis under by tightening your buttocks and abdominal muscles. (Rock your pelvis forward.)

★ **7. Start:** Stand with your feet hip-width apart, knees loose, hands on your hips.

7a. *Gently* arch your lower back. (Rock backward.)

7b. Tuck your pelvis under by tightening your buttocks and abdominal muscles. (Rock forward.)

★ **8. Start:** Lie on your back on the floor with both knees bent.

8a. *Gently* arch your lower back off the floor. (Rock backward.)

8b. Tuck your pelvis under and flatten your lower back by tightening your buttocks and abdominal muscles. (Rock forward.)

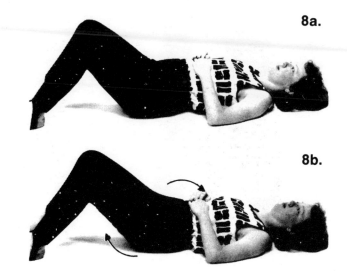

51

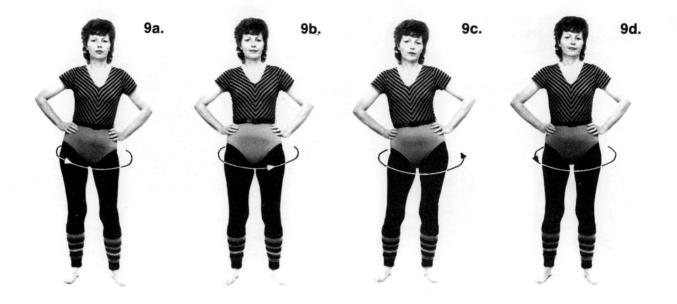

9a.   9b.   9c.   9d.

10.

9. Start: Stand with your feet hip-width apart, hands on your hips. Keep your knees loose.

Caution: Do this exercise very carefully if you have sciatica or a severe back condition.

9a–d. Roll your pelvis around in a circle, taking it sideways, forwards, to the other side and backwards. Move from your waist and keep your upper body still. Roll your pelvis around in the other direction.

10. Start: Stand with your feet apart and hands on your waist.

Keeping both feet flat, stretch one arm up and across your body. Let your body twist and look at your hand. Repeat to the other side.

★ **11. Start:** Lie on your back with your knees bent and hands on your thighs.

Caution: If you have problems with your neck, use a pillow.

Tuck your chin in. Lift your shoulders by sliding your hands up towards your knees. Lower slowly, keeping your chin tucked in.

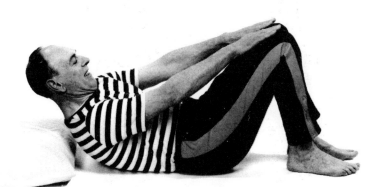

12. Start: Lie on your back with your knees bent and your feet apart.

Caution: If you have problems with your neck, use a pillow.

Tuck your chin in and lift your shoulders to one side by sliding both hands up towards one knee. Lower slowly, keeping your chin tucked in. Repeat to the other side.

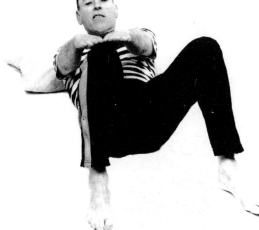

13a. Start: Lie on your back with both knees bent up towards your chest. Stretch both arms out sideways.

Caution: Do not do this exercise if you have had a hip replacement.

13b. Take both knees over to one side. *Do not* go further than half-way to the floor. Repeat to the other side.

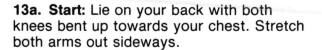

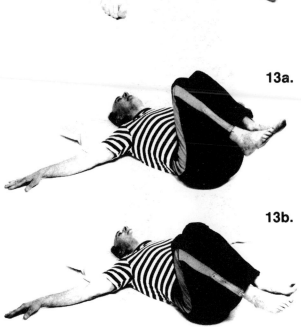

13a.

13b.

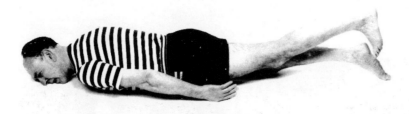

14. Start: Lie on your front with your hands by your sides.

Lift one leg up off the floor, with the knee straight. Keep both front hip bones on the floor.

15. Start: Lie on your back with your knees bent up towards your chest and your hands on your knees.

Caution: Take care with this exercise if you have a hip replacement.

Massage your lower back by gently rocking your pelvis around in small circles. Circle in both directions.

15a.

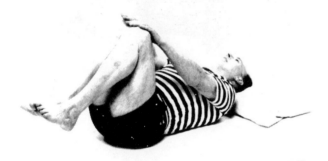

15b.

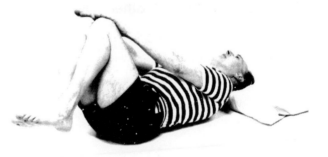

15c.

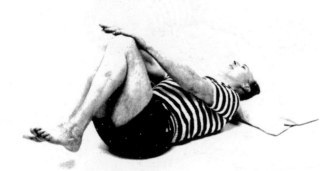

15d.

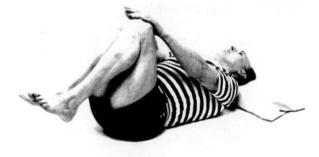

16a.   **16b.**

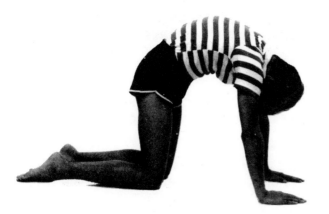

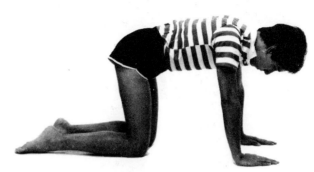

Caution: *Do not do Exercises 16–21 if you have shoulder, wrist or knee problems.*

16. Start: On hands and knees with your hands under your shoulders and your knees under your hips.

16a. Tuck under your head and your tail, and arch upwards with your back.

16b. Lower slowly and *flatten* your back. Do not let your back arch downwards.

17. Start: On hands and knees.

Without moving your head, 'wag your tail' from side to side. Do not arch your back.

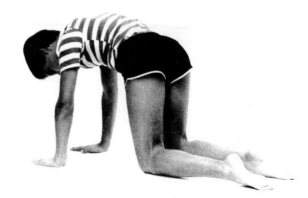

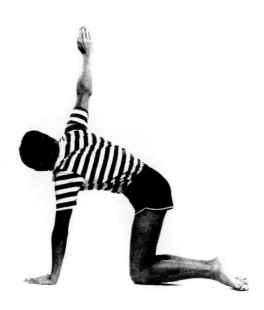

Caution:
The following exercises are specifically for people with ankylosing spondylitis. Take care if you have other back conditions.

18. Start: On your hands and knees with your hands under your shoulders and knees under your hips.

Look at one hand as you lift it out to the side and upwards, letting your spine twist.

19. Start: On your hands and knees.

Without moving your hands, stretch your bottom back towards your heels. Hold the stretch for about 5 seconds.

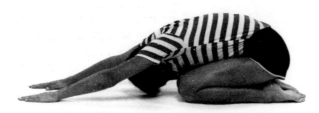

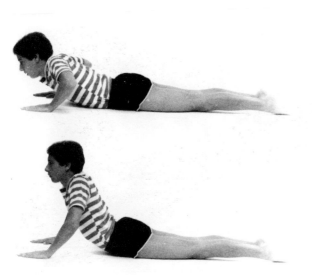

20. Start: Lie on your front with your hands under your shoulders.

Lift up your head and then push up through your hands to lift your *shoulders only*. Keep your chest on the floor. Hold for a few seconds before lowering slowly.

21. Start: Lie on your front with your hands under your shoulders.

Lift up your head and then push up through your hands and lift up your chest. Keep your front hip-bones on the floor. Hold for a few seconds before lowering slowly.

HIPS

The hip joint is a ball and socket joint — made up of a ball part on the end of the thigh bone which fits into a curved socket in the pelvis. It is a joint which needs a large range of movement, combined with the strength and stability required to bear the weight of your body. The joint is well supported by those large strong muscles of your upper and outer thighs and your buttocks.

The hip is a common site for arthritis, both osteoarthritis and rheumatoid arthritis. You may feel the pain from an arthritic hip in the groin or the upper or outer thigh, or even referred down to the knee or below. If you have arthritis in your hip, you need to build up the strength of the muscles supporting it. You have to keep mobile too, so you can put on your socks and tie your shoelaces.

Nowadays, complete hip replacements are quite common and usually very successful.

This may be a solution if your hip pain is chronic and severe. If you have had a hip replacement, it's very important that you strengthen the muscles which provide support for your hip. There are, however, some movements which you must avoid because they endanger the stability of your artificial hip. You should not bend your hip more than 90°, and you should not cross the leg with the hip replacement over in front of your other leg. One of the worst things you can do is to sit with your legs crossed!

If you have a hip replacement, take note of the cautions on Exercises 1 and 4.

If you have difficulty getting down onto the floor, just do the sitting and standing exercises.

Start by doing 2–4 of each exercise.
Key hip exercises: 3, 4, 7.

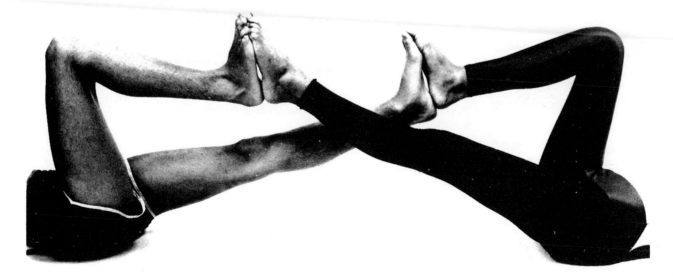

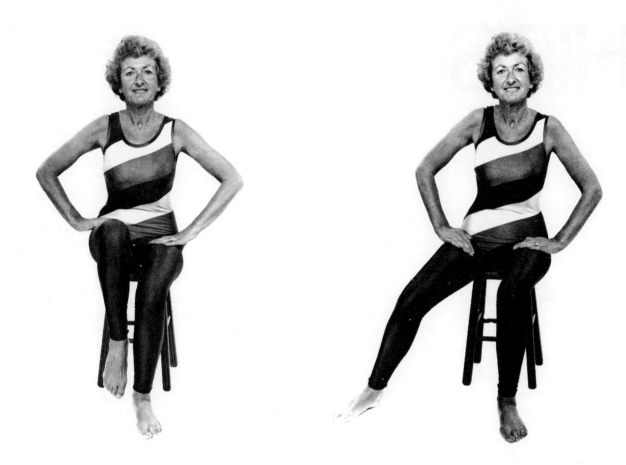

1. Start: Sit on a chair with both feet on the floor.

Caution: Be careful if you have a hip replacement.

Keep your back straight and lift up one knee. Lower slowly, then repeat with the other leg.

2. Start: Sit with your feet flat.

Keep your body still and lift one leg out to the side, then back in. Repeat with the other leg.

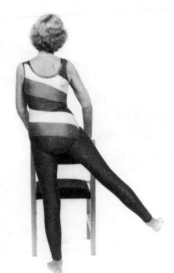

★ **3. Start:** Stand, holding onto the back of a chair with both hands.

Keep your body upright as you lift one leg out to the side, with your foot flexed and toes pointing forward. Lower slowly and repeat with the other leg.

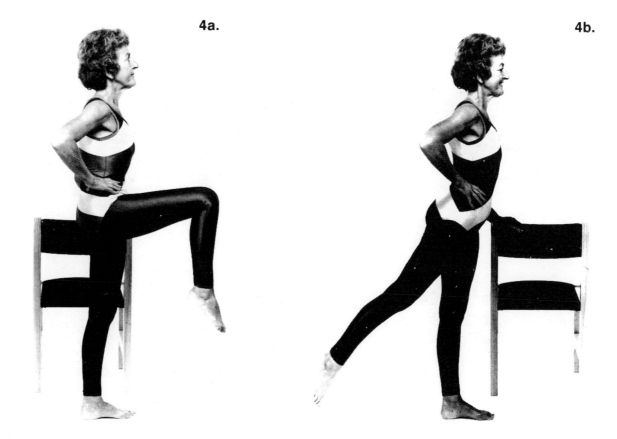

4a. **4b.**

★ **4. Start:** Stand, holding onto the back of a chair with one hand.

Caution: Do not lift any part of your leg above hip level if you have a hip replacement.

4a. Keep your back straight and lift up your outside knee.

4b. Straighten your knee as you stretch your leg behind you, with your toes just off the floor. Turn around to work the other leg.

5. Start: Lie on your back with your legs out straight.

Keep your leg straight and your toes pointing upwards. Slide one leg out to the side and then back in. Repeat with the other leg.

5.

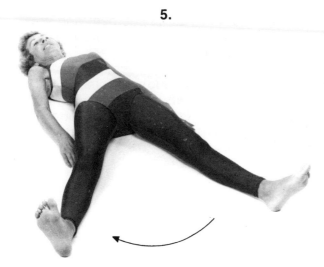

6a.　　　　　　　　　　　　　　　　　　　　　**6b.**

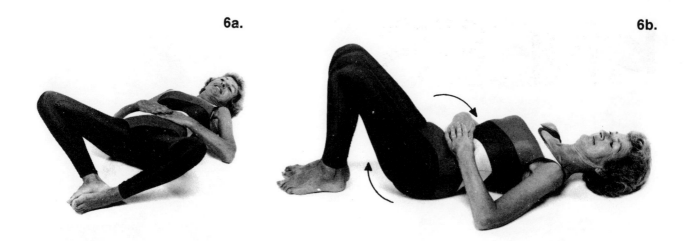

6. Start: Lie on your back with your knees bent and your feet together.

6a. Keep your feet together and slowly stretch your knees apart.

6b. Close your knees and press them together as you tilt your pelvis upwards (refer back exercises 6–8) — tighten your buttocks and your stomach muscles.

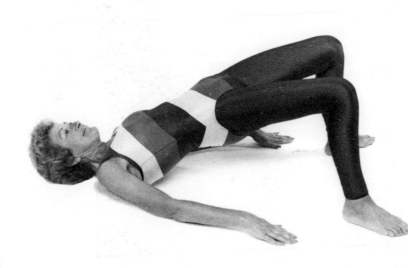

★**7. Start:** Lie on your back with your knees bent and your feet and knees comfortably apart.

Push through your feet and slowly lift your bottom off the floor. Lower slowly, rolling your spine onto the floor from the top downwards.

KNEES

The knee is a common problem site for people with arthritis — both osteoarthritis and rheumatoid arthritis. The knee joint acts like a hinge — it can only bend and straighten. It needs to be strong since it is being used constantly during normal daily activities. The knee acts as one of the main shock absorbers for the jarring which occurs each time we take a step.

The large muscle in the front of your thigh is known as the quadriceps muscle. It is this muscle which straightens and supports your knee and holds you upright. Therefore it is crucial that this muscle is strong. If your knees feel weak or give way, then concentrate on Exercises 1, 2 and 7 which will strengthen the quadriceps muscle.

Arthritic knees can sometimes look a bit unsightly. They may become large and puffy-looking or you may be knock-kneed or bow-legged. This does not mean that they have to be less functional, though. Some people are unable to straighten their knees completely or they may have unstable wobbly joints.

If your knees have any of these problems, concentrate on strengthening the quadriceps muscles to give your knees as much support as possible (Exercises 1, 2 and 7).

If you have particularly painful or unstable knees, omit Exercises 4, 5 and 6: they may put too much strain on your knees.

Knee replacements are becoming more common these days. If you have a knee replacement, you should not try to bend your knee beyond 90° as this may overstrain the joint. Note the caution in Exercise 8.

Good supportive shoes with a cushioned sole will help if you have knee problems. They will absorb some of the jarring which is normally passed on through the knee with every step you take.

Start with 2–4 repetitions of each exercise.

Key exercises: 2, 7.

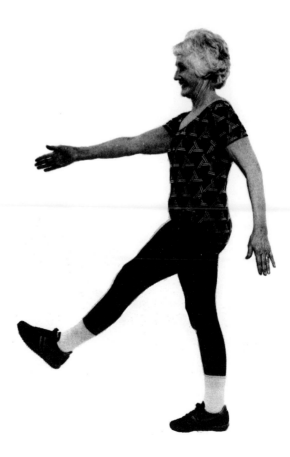

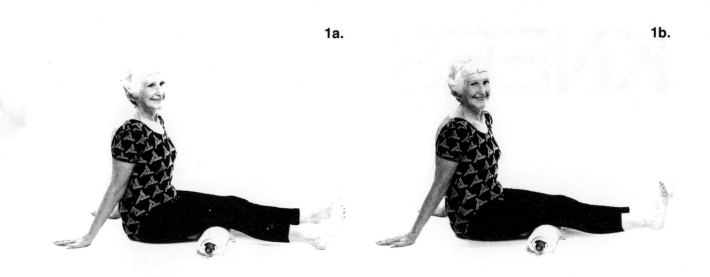

1a. (top left image)

1b. (top right image)

1a. Start: Sit or lie on the floor with your legs out straight. Wrap a rolling pin in a towel. Place it under one leg just above the crease of your knee.

1b. Flex your foot back. Straighten your knee by pushing down onto the towel and lifting your heel. Hold for 3–5 seconds, then lower slowly.

★ **2. Start:** Sit up straight on a chair with your thighs fully supported.

Flex your foot back and straighten your knee. Keep your back straight and your thigh on the chair. Hold for 3–5 seconds, then lower slowly.

3. Start: Sit up straight about half-way to the edge of the chair.

Extend one foot forward onto its heel and bend the other foot backward onto its toes. Change legs.

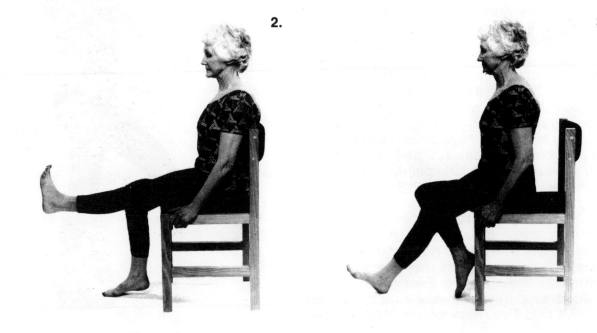

4. Start: Stand, holding the back of a chair with both hands.

Keep your knees together and bend one knee by lifting your foot backwards. Lower slowly.

5. Start: Stand with your feet hip-width apart, toes facing forward. Hold the back of a chair for support.

Caution: Take care if you have severe knee problems.

Keep your back straight and slowly bend your knees *over your toes*. Straighten, by pushing up through your feet.

6. Start: Stand with your feet comfortably apart, your toes turned slightly outwards. Hold the back of a chair if you need support.

Caution: Take care if you have severe knee problems.

Keep your back straight and slowly bend your knees *over your toes*. Straighten, by pushing up through your feet.

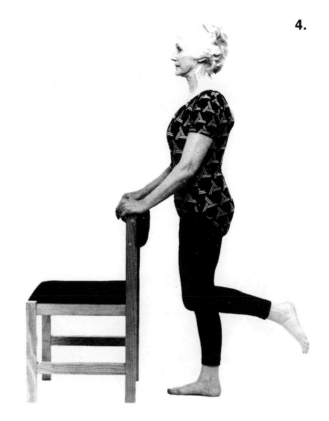

4.

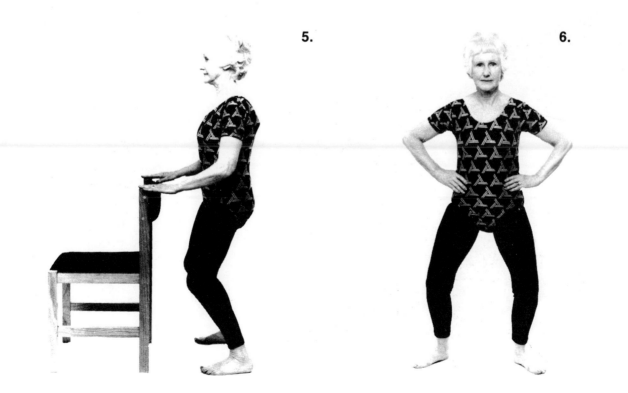

5.

6.

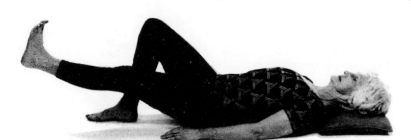

★**7. Start:** Lie on your back with one leg bent.

Flex back the foot and tighten your knee. Lift your straight leg about 60 cm (2 ft) off the floor. Lower slowly, touching the floor with your calf first.

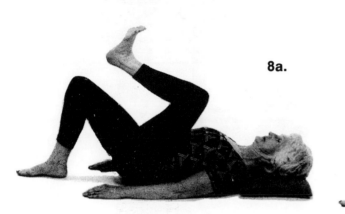

8a.

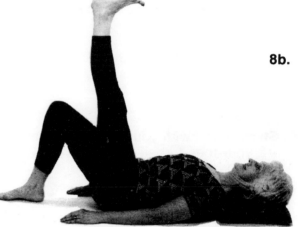

8b.

8. Start: Lie on your back with one leg bent.

Caution: Take care with this exercise if you have a hip or knee replacement. Do not bend your hip or knee beyond 90°.

8a. Bend the knee of the straight leg up towards your chest.

8b–d. Straighten your leg by pushing out with your heel. Bend your leg again, then push out at a different level. Extend at 3–5 different levels.

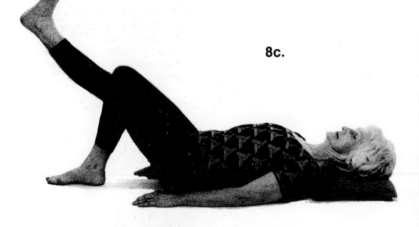

8c.

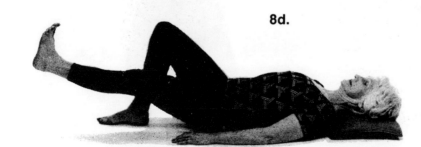

8d.

FEET

Our feet do so much wonderful work for us —
and we so often neglect or abuse them.

The best way to look after your feet is by
wearing suitable footwear. Not only will good
shoes protect and support them, but they will
also cushion your feet and knees to some
extent. For everyday wear, choose shoes with
rounded toes, a flattish heel and support for
the instep. You should be able to move your
toes inside your shoes. Another important
feature is a shock-absorbing heel and sole.
Good quality jogging shoes are perfect not
only for jogging but also for everyday wear —
particularly if you spend a lot of time on your
feet or like to go walking.

The ankle joint may become inflamed with
rheumatoid arthritis or may develop osteoarthritis following a bad ankle injury. Also the
ligaments and tendons supporting the joint
can easily be 'sprained'. So strengthening
the muscles will help support and stabilize
the ankle.

The natural arch, or instep, of the foot plays
a vital role in keeping us balanced on our feet
and in absorbing some of the shock of
walking. If you have 'fallen arches', more
stress is put onto the bones across the ball of
your foot. This can be quite a common site for
arthritis. Exercise 4 helps to strengthen the
arches of the foot. If your ankles or feet are
very painful, do not do the weight-bearing
Exercises 6–9.

Start with 2–4 of each exercise.
Key exercises: 1, 2, 4.

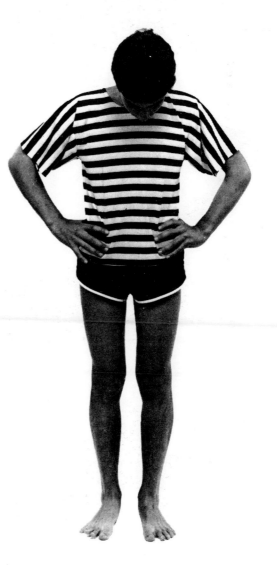

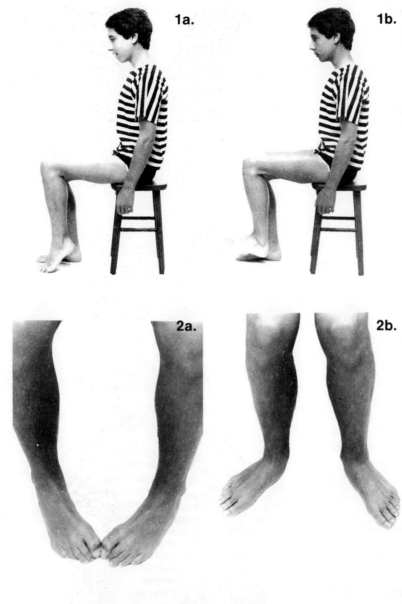

1a.

1b.

★**1. Start:** Sit with both feet flat.

1a. Lift the heel of one foot, leaving the ball of your foot on the floor.

1b. Lift up your entire foot by bending it up at the ankle. Lower onto the ball of your foot and then onto your heel. Repeat with the other foot.

2a.

2b.

★**2. Start:** Sit with both feet flat and slightly apart.

2a. Without moving your heels, turn the soles of your feet in towards each other.

2b. Without moving your heels, turn the soles of your feet away from each other.

3. Start: Sit with one foot lifted just off the floor.

3a–d. Rotate your foot from the ankle, making a circle with your big toe. Circle the other way.

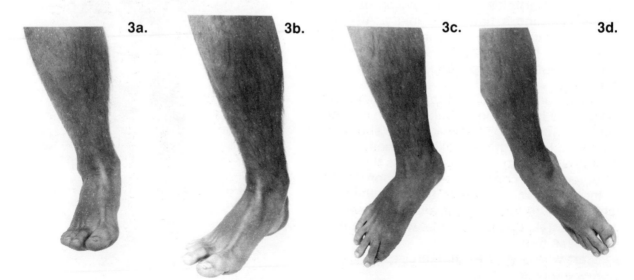

3a.

3b.

3c.

3d.

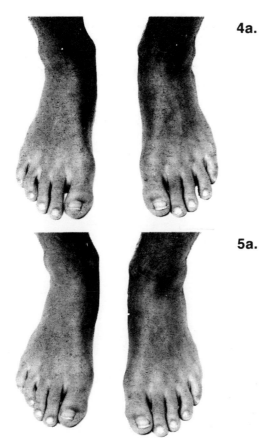

4a.   **4b.**

5a.   **5b.**

★ **4a. Start:** Sit with your feet flat on the floor.

4b. Keep your heels and toes on the floor and lift the arches on the inside of your feet.

5a. Start: Sit with your feet flat on the floor.

5b. Spread your toes apart and then relax. Keep persevering.

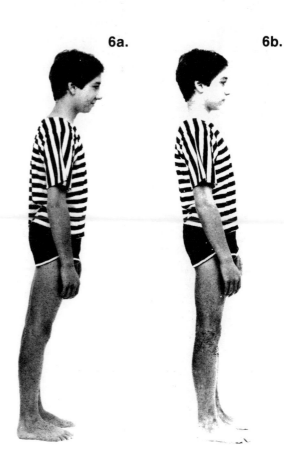

6a.   **6b.**

6. Start: Stand up straight with your feet together, toes pointing forward.

6a. Keep your body stiff and your feet flat; sway your weight forward.

6b. Sway your weight backward, keeping your body stiff.

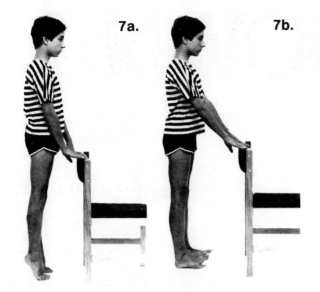

7a.   **7b.**

7. Start: Stand with your feet together, holding the back of a chair.

Caution: Take care if you have severe ankle or foot problems.

7a. Push up onto your toes.

7b. Lower slowly and then rock back onto your heels and lift your toes.

8a.   **8b.**

8. Start: Stand with your feet together, holding the back of a chair.

Caution: Take care if you have severe ankle or foot problems.

8a. Push up onto your toes.

8b. Slowly lower one heel. Rise up onto your toes again, then lower the other heel.

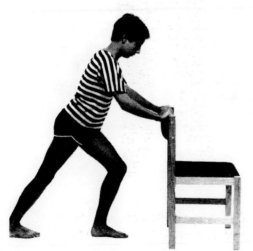

9. Start: Stand with one foot behind the other, both feet facing straight forward. Hold a chair for support.

Keep both heels on the floor as you bend your front knee forward. Keep your back knee straight. Stop when you feel a stretch in the calf of your back leg. Hold the stretch for 3–5 seconds and then slowly release.

COOL DOWN

The purpose of the cool down is to provide a pleasant relaxing completion to your exercise routine. Just as it was necessary to warm up your joints and muscles before doing more strenuous exercises, it is also good to reintegrate your body afterwards.

This cool-down exercise combines breathing with movement and should be performed slowly, smoothly, and meditatively. You can sit or stand to do the exercise.

Start by just learning the movement sequence, then begin to combine the breathing with the movements. Once you know what you are doing, think about the quality — let each movement roll smoothly into the next — feel that each movement 'floats' on your breath so that you are moving and breathing together.

This exercise can be done at any time during the day if you are feeling a bit uptight — its meditative quality will help you to relax.

Repeat the whole sequence 2–4 times.

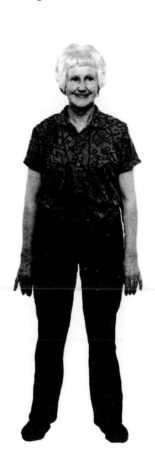

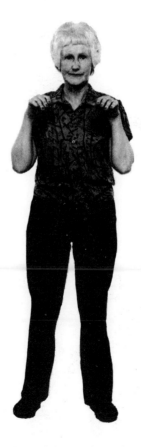

1. Start: Sit or stand with your feet comfortably apart and your arms by your sides. Take a slow breath *in and out*.

2. *Breathe in* as you lift your wrists up to your shoulders, keeping your hands relaxed.

3.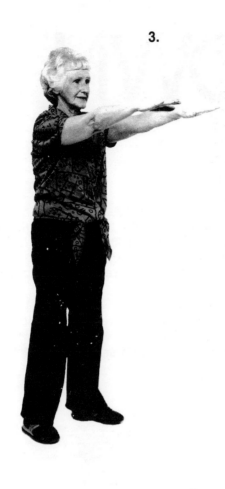

4.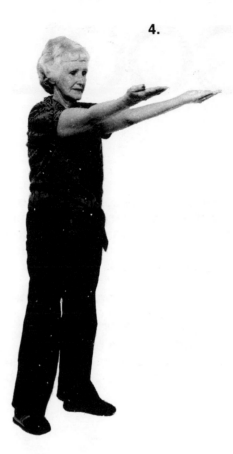

5.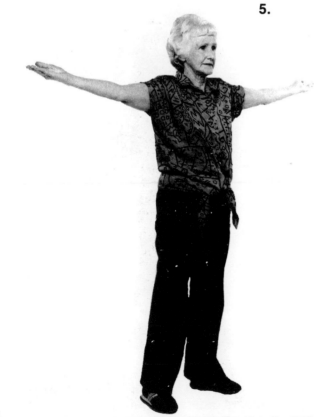

3. *Breathe out* as you stretch both arms forward, palms down.

4. Turn your palms upwards.

5. *Breathe in* as you open your arms out to the sides, palms upward.

6. Turn your palms down.

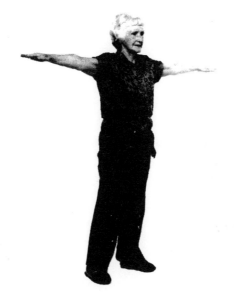

7. *Breathe out* as you swing your arms down and across your body.

8. *Breathe in* as you lift your arms out to the side.

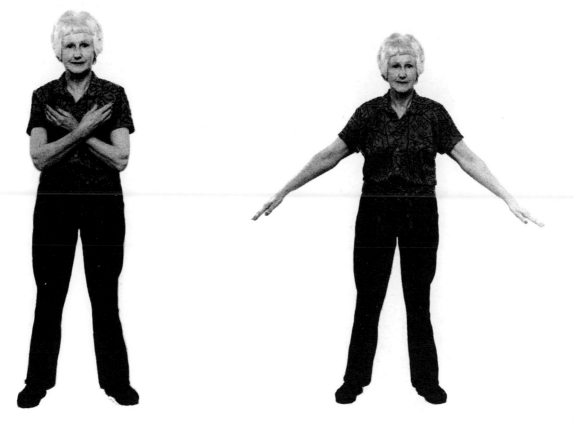

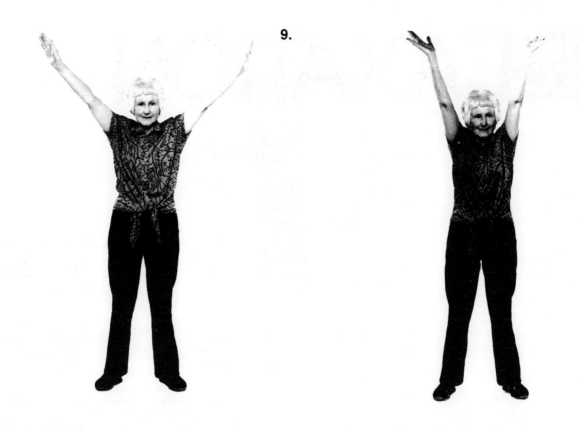

9.

10.

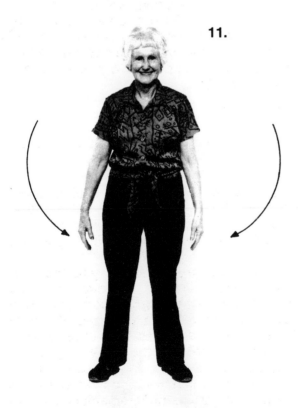

11.

9. Stretch your arms above your head.

10. Give an extra stretch by pushing upwards with the palms of your hands.

11. *Breathe out* as you lower your arms sideways and return to your starting position.

Repeat movements 1–11 a few times.

RELAXATION

For some of us, relaxation is the most difficult exercise of all. It is easy to say to someone else, 'Don't worry about it. Just relax.' But when we are dealing with our own pain or our own problems and worries, it's a different matter. We find that relaxation does not always come easily.

Whether you have arthritis or not, relaxation is one of the most important exercises you can ever learn. If you do have arthritis, you are no doubt aware that it causes you more trouble when you are upset or under stress. It may seem that you experience more pain, or maybe it's just that you are less able to cope with it.

The connection also works the other way. Prolonged pain can be very depressing and often creates inner tension. With arthritis also, the muscles surrounding a joint may tense up to prevent any movement which may cause pain. This close interaction between pain and tension can result in a downward spiral in which pain causes tension . . . causes more pain . . . causes more tension . . . and so on!

If you want to start coming up again, you have to break the cycle by reducing either your pain or your tension. We know pain can be relieved by the use of comfort techniques (refer page 13) or by appropriate medication. But relaxation is very helpful in reducing your general level of tension, both physical and mental. By lessening your general tension, you are able to cope much better with your level of pain.

There are a number of techniques you can use to develop a sense of deep relaxation. We will describe some of these. Remember, though, that relaxation is like any other skill. Practice is the key to success. This means that you should do these exercises regularly, not just when you are feeling uptight.

Relaxation is a natural complement to physical activity. Regular physical exercise works the muscles of the body and so helps to release general muscle tension. A good time to practice your relaxation is just after you have completed your workout.

METHODS OF RELAXATION

First, a number of 'quick and easy' ways to relax — yawning, laughing, sighing, stretching or shaking various parts or all your body, doing the cool-down exercise (page 69).

Certain activities that don't require a lot of concentration can be very relaxing. Perhaps you enjoy reading, knitting, walking along the beach, listening to music, working in the garden.

You might like to relieve your muscle tension by soaking in a hot bath or spa or by treating yourself to a massage. What bliss!

All these suggestions are useful; but a deeper form of relaxation, which quiets your mind as well as releases tension from your body, is more beneficial. You need about 15-20 minutes in which to practice these deep relaxation techniques, so choose a time when you will be undisturbed.

We have included a number of different techniques for you to try. You will find that some work for you better than others. Try them all, then choose the methods you find most beneficial.

For the first few sessions, you may not achieve deep relaxation. You may think you have failed to do the exercise correctly. But if you are very tense or in a lot of pain, it's more difficult to achieve a deep level of relaxation. The more you practice the easier it gets.

It is well worth persevering because it's in these situations that you have most need of relaxation. What you must remember is *not to try* too hard. Relaxation will come of its own accord if you can adopt a passive attitude without too many expectations.

73

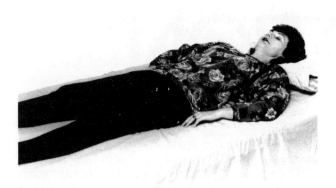

Lie on your back with a low pillow under your head. Have your legs slightly apart and let your feet fall outwards. Rest your arms by your sides.

Relaxation Positions

Before you start, make sure your body is comfortable and fully supported. It is best to lie on the floor or a firm bed with a low pillow for your head. A chair is all right provided it gives your body good support, preferably with a head rest.

Three lying positions are shown. Try these or find another position in which you feel comfortable. Keep warm throughout your relaxation session. As your body becomes more relaxed it cools down, so cover yourself with a light rug, particularly if you have been exercising. Be sure that your clothing is not restrictive. Loosen anything that is tight around your body. Take off your shoes.

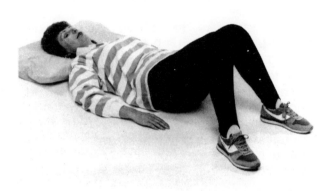

Lie on your back with a low pillow under your head. Bend up both legs so your feet are comfortably apart and your knees rest together. This is a good position if you have low back pain.

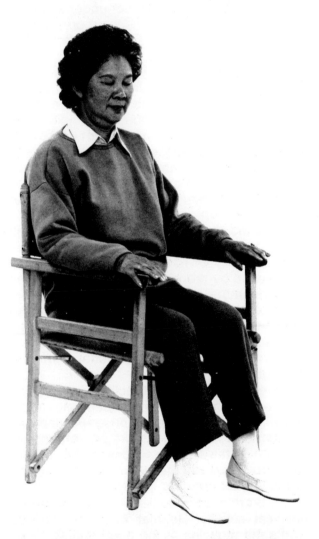

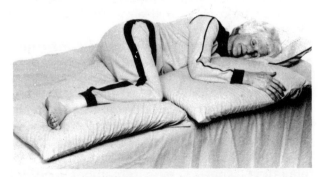

Lie on your side with a low pillow under your head. Rest your top arm and leg forward on to pillows.

Sit well back into a chair with your thighs supported and your feet flat on the floor.

Technique 1: Concentration on Breathing

Lie down in your comfortable supported position. As you lie there, become aware of your breath. Follow the air as you breathe in and breathe out. Allow your breath to flow easily and evenly. Don't try to force yourself to take deep breaths. After a short time, start to count each breath silently as you breathe out. Begin with the first breath out as 'one' and continue up to 'ten'. Then start again at 'one'. If you find yourself drifting off into other thoughts, don't worry. Just start again by counting 'one' with your next breath. It doesn't matter if you lose count or repeat numbers. The counting is only a way of focussing your mind. It's not significant in itself.

Keep concentrating on your breathing for about 10–15 minutes. You can open your eyes occasionally to look at the clock, but position it so that you don't have to move your head. Experience and enjoy the feeling of relaxation for a short time before you think about getting up. When you are ready, move and stretch a little, then open your eyes and *slowly* sit up.

Technique 2: Breathing into Various Parts of the Body

Settle into a comfortable position and then concentrate on your breath. Allow it to flow evenly and rhythmically, without force. Concentrate on your *out-breath*. Imagine that with each breath out you are releasing stored up tensions from your body. Don't think about the in-breath. It will take care of itself.

After about 10 of these breaths, imagine that you are breathing out through various parts of your body. As your breath flows through, it releases the tension from that part of your body. Imagine 'breathing out' through your right leg . . . your left leg . . . your pelvic area . . . your stomach . . . your right arm . . . your left arm . . . between your shoulder blades . . . down your back . . . over your face . . . and through your hair. Send 2–3 breaths to each body region and then spend some time on your problem area. Imagine that your breath is warm and soothing. Imagine that, as it flows through your arthritic joints, it relieves the pain and releases the tension in the surrounding muscles.

Finish by enjoying the sense of peace and relaxation you have produced in your body.

Gradually come back by moving and stretching a little, opening your eyes and then slowly getting up.

These are just a few ways in which you can learn to experience relaxation. You can learn other relaxation techniques at yoga and meditation classes or stress management courses. There are books you can read and also some relaxation tapes available which talk you through your relaxation session.

Try to practice relaxation 3–4 times each week. After a while the feeling of deep relaxation comes much more easily. You will soon discover that you can use the techniques effectively when you are tense or in pain. Perhaps it will dawn on you that you are generally less tense and better able to cope with your pain. Remember, relaxation is another means which can help you manage your arthritis. The power of the mind is very strong. Regular deep relaxation can reduce or replace your reliance on pain medication.

RELAXATION AND SLEEP

Maybe you fell asleep during or after a relaxation session. That's fine. It means you were truly relaxed. If you do not sleep well during the night, this is a good opportunity to catch up on some sleep. Painful joints often make undisturbed sleep difficult if you have arthritis. By resting and sleeping for a while during the day, you'll need less sleep during the night.

General tiredness is a common problem for people with arthritis, particularly rheumatoid arthritis. If you do get weary during the day, listen to your body. Plan your daily activities so you can have a half hour to one hour rest period. This may make the difference between coping and not coping with the rest of the day.

You can try these techniques at night whenever you have difficulty getting off to sleep, or when you wake up during the night. In this situation, the same thoughts may keep circling around and around in your head. You need to break this cycle by focusing your thoughts in a different direction. All the techniques described above can be useful in refocusing and quieting your thoughts. Select the technique with which you are most comfortable. Try it next time you are having trouble finding those sweet dreams.

USING YOUR BODY

POSTURE

Were you often told to 'sit up straight'? Well, good posture not only makes you look better, but it also puts less strain on your joints. Maintaining good posture does not just mean standing or sitting in the 'correct' position. Posture is a dynamic activity, so you need to be just as aware of it when you are moving as when you are still.

Have you noticed what happens to your posture when you are feeling 'on top of the world' compared to when you are feeling 'down in the dumps'? Our emotions are expressed in the way we sit, stand and move. It can work the other way too. By lifting your body you help to lift your spirits.

Of course, it's a lot easier to sag and slump rather than make the effort to maintain good posture. But have you forgotten that one of the functions of muscles is to take some of the strain off the joints? By slouching, you are hanging the weight of your body onto the ligaments and other structures surrounding the joints. This can put extra stress on an already damaged joint. But the other extreme is just about as bad — using a lot of muscular effort trying to hold a straight rigid posture. This will just make your joints feel stiffer.

Good posture is the result of a dynamic balance of muscular forces. It essentially relies on good tone in the postural muscles. As you continue with your exercise program, you will find that your posture improves automatically.

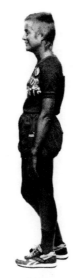

Bad posture — standing

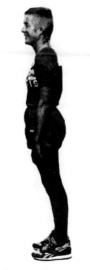

Good posture — standing

77

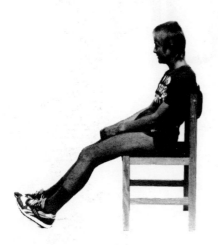

Bad posture — sitting

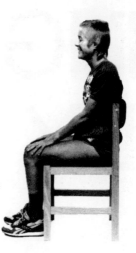

Good posture — sitting

The best way to align your body correctly is to imagine that the crown of your head is attached by a string to a balloon and that the rest of your body is suspended from it. Think of being lifted up through the central axis of your body. When you apply this concept, you will find that your back and neck lengthen and straighten, your shoulders drop and fall back, your chest lifts, your tummy flattens and your buttocks tuck under. Just watch that you have not also lifted your chin. It ought to remain slightly dropped because you are lifting through the *crown* of your head (refer neck Exercise 2, page 35).

Look at yourself in a mirror and see the difference. But be conscious that this is not a static position. Try to think of that balloon when you are walking or doing your exercises, and throughout all your other daily activities.

Sitting posture is important, too. We spend so much of our life in chairs. Many modern chairs seem to encourage us to sink into them, and it is virtually impossible to maintain a good sitting posture. Not only are they difficult to get out of, but often they do not give very good support to your body and soon become quite uncomfortable.

The ideal comfortable chair allows you to sit with your bottom back in the chair — your thighs fully supported and your feet flat on the floor. The back of the chair should offer firm support right along your spine. It is useful to have arm rests.

Of course, you can still think of the balloon holding you up when you are sitting. Slumping in a chair will eventually lead to low back-

ache because of the strain being put on the ligaments and muscles of the lumbar or lower spine. A small cushion placed behind your lower back often relieves backache. This is a particularly useful item for long car journeys since many car seats are not very supportive.

Key exercises for posture:
Warm Up 5
Neck 2
Neck 6
Back 1
Back 6, 7, 8
Feet 6

LIFTING

Lifting incorrectly puts a great strain on your lower back. *Do not bend over* when you want

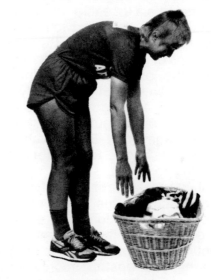

Lifting — incorrect method

78

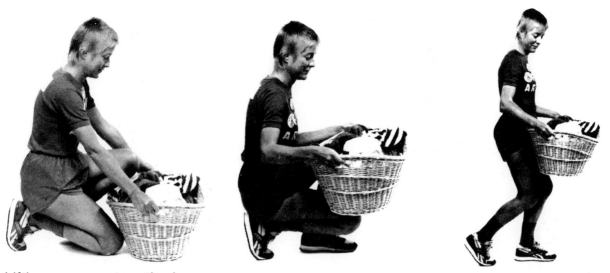

Lifting — correct method

to lift something up from the floor or ground, or take something out from a low cupboard or shelf. Instead, you should use the strong muscles of your legs to do the work.

So, when lifting, always try to follow this sequence:
1. Bend your knees and squat down close to the object you want to lift.
2. Lift the object and hold it close to your body.
3. Keep your *back straight* and stand up by *straightening your knees*.

The only problem with this method is that it does put a strain on your knees. If you have pain in your knee, use your mouth to lift heavy objects — ask someone else! You don't want to have an injured back as well as a bad knee!

USEFUL ADDRESSES

The Arthritis Foundation provides information, newsletters, and literature to those who suffer from any form of arthritis. In addition, the Arthritis Foundation has many regional chapters throughout the United States and Canada that can provide assistance on a local level. To obtain information about the Arthritis Foundation or one of its chapters, contact:

Arthritis Foundation (National Office)
1314 Spring Street N.W.
Atlanta, Georgia 30309

(404) 872-7100

Another group that provides information about dealing with chronic pain is the National Chronic Pain Outreach, a nonprofit organization staffed by volunteers. This group may also be able to provide the names of chronic pain support groups in you area. Contact them at:

National Chronic Pain Outreach
4922 Hampden Lane
Bethesda, Maryland 20814

(301) 652-4948

FURTHER READING

Fries, J.F. *Arthritis: A Comprehensive Guide*. Reading, MA: Addison-Wesley, 1986.

Krewer, S., and Edgar A. *The Arthritis Exercise Book*. New York: Cornerstone Library, 1981.

Lazarus, A. *In the Mind's Eye*. New York: Rawson Associates, 1977.

Linchitz, R. *Life Without Pain*. Reading, MA: Addison-Wesley, 1988.

Lorig, K., and Fries, J.F. *The Arthritis Helpbook*. rev. ed. Reading, MA: Addison-Wesley, 1986.

Phillips, R. *Coping With Rheumatoid Arthritis*. Garden City Park, NY: Avery Publishing Group, 1988.

Phillips, R. *Coping With Osteoarthritis*. Garden City Park, NY: Avery Publishing Group, 1989.

INDEX

Joint
    effects of ankylosing spondylitis, 7
    effects of osteoarthritis, 6
    effects of rheumatoid arthritis, 4, 5
    pain relief, 11, 12–13. *See also* Treatment.
    structure of, 3–4
Joint capsule, 4

Knees, exercises for, 24, 32, 61–64

Lifting, 78
Ligaments, 4
Lumbar spondylosis, 6. *See also* Osteo-
    arthritis.

Medication, 11–12. *See also* Treatment.
Muscles, 4

Neck, exercises for, 33–36
Non-steroidal anti-inflammatory drugs, 11

OA. *See* Osteoarthritis.
Occupational therapist, 12
Osteoarthritis
    causes of, 6
    definition, 6
    effects of, 6
    exercises for, 7, 43–45, 48–56, 57–60, 61–
    64. *See also* specific body parts.
    onset of, 6
    prognosis, 7
    who it affects, 7
Osteoarthrosis. *See* Osteoarthritis.
Osteophytes, 6
Osteoporosis, 8

Penicillamine, 12
Physical therapy, 12
Physician, 10–11, *See also* Treatment.
Posture, 77–78
Pyramid Food Plan, 9–10

Quadriceps muscle, 61

Relaxation techniques, 73–75
Rheumatism, 8
Rheumatoid arthritis
    causes, 5
    definition, 4
    effects of, 5
    exercises for, 5–6, 21–26, 37–42, 43–45,
    57–60. *See also* specific body parts.
    onset of, 4
    prognosis, 4–5
    who it affects, 4

Stress, 10
Surgery, 12
Synovial fluid, 4, 6
Synovial membrane, 4, 5

Tendon, 4
Tendonitis, 8
Treatment, 11–13
    doctor, 10–11
    medication, 11–12
    mental attitude, 10
    occupational therapy, 12
    physical therapy, 12
    surgery, 12

Weather, effects on arthritis, 13